THE
SHOT

THE HARROWING JOURNEY
OF A MARINE IN
THE WAR ON TERROR

BILL BEE and WILLS ROBINSON

KNOX
K
PRESS

A KNOX PRESS BOOK
An Imprint of Permuted Press
ISBN: 978-1-63758-301-2
ISBN (eBook): 978-1-63758-302-9

The Shot:
The Harrowing Journey of a Marine in the War on Terror

Cover photo by Goran Tomasevic/Reuters
Cover art by Cody Corcoran

This is a work of nonfiction. All people, locations, events, and situations are portrayed to the best of the author's memory.

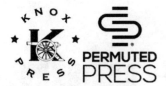

Permuted Press, LLC
New York • Nashville
permutedpress.com

Published in the United States of America

1 2 3 4 5 6 7 8 9 10

CHAPTER 1

It was around 115 degrees in Helmand Province, on May 18, 2008, the day of the shot that would cement my place in the history of the War on Terror.

I was inside a hole that a mouse would have struggled to survive in. I was twenty-six years old on my third deployment in Afghanistan, the sweaty asshole of the world. It was like living in an Easy Bake Oven made of dirt. Mutant ants with gigantic legs were scurrying everywhere and crawling into my pants and bag packed with ammo and gear. Between the bugs and months without a shower, I had been constantly scratching my legs, and I couldn't remember the last time I had enjoyed a hint of comfort: a bed sheet, a couch, the sound of a female voice.

I was gazing into the sun and dreaming of my wife Bobbie cradling her pregnant belly, and our unborn son 7,420 miles away in Johnstown, Pennsylvania, when I felt the single shot fly just a few feet above my head.

The sound of a round cutting through the silky heat waves at high speed was something I had become too familiar with as a Marine. I could tell it was a round from either a Soviet-era SKS semi-automatic rifle or a Dragunov sniper, fired by a Taliban marksman who had our platoon in his sights. But I couldn't see him. The terrorists were experts in hiding.

I got ready to move. I knew the drill. From the moment our platoon set foot in Garmsir, we had been sucked into three or four major firefights a day. They were so regular we learned to sleep through them. Hundreds of Marines who had just left high school, and were barely old enough to buy a six-pack of beer, were using M203 grenade launchers attached to M16A4 rifles—among the most lethal in the world—to fight one of the biggest Taliban insurgencies since the invasion in 2001.

I was a squad leader in 4th Platoon, Alpha Company in 1st Battalion, 6th Marines, set up in the tiny compound where we had been living for almost a week. It was one of the many mud huts in Garmsir we had taken position in, during our month away from Kandahar Airfield, to help British forces drive the extremists out.

When the sniper took aim at me and my men, I had just been relieved from a four-hour watch rotation as Sergeant of the Guard. I was trying to enjoy the little bit of downtime by washing the only extra T-shirt and pair of green silkies I had, with my grunt version of a washer-dryer: a hand-operated water pump, laundry detergent I found when we raided a building, and an old, rusty bucket to rinse. Looking at the brown water, I thought this could only be making my clothes dirtier. But it was a chore that made life seem somewhat normal, if only for a few minutes.

I dropped my dirty clothes when I heard the shot. Every second was crucial, and a delay or mistake would almost certainly mean people in my squad—or I—would die. The round brought with it a rush of adrenaline, igniting my muscle memory built from hours of drills outside Camp Lejeune in North Carolina. No matter how many times it happens, the sound of a round cracking over you will always quicken the pulse.

I crouched down and grabbed my M16A4 rifle, which was already loaded with a magazine and ready to unleash hell. The gun is light, easy to carry, helps Marines run into positions as quickly as possible, and has a deadly precision that I constantly prayed I could use on a target. I had spent eight years dedicated to that rifle, and fired hundreds of thousands of rounds preparing to engage with the enemy. The last time was just the day before, in another firefight with a Taliban unit just a couple of hundred yards away, and I couldn't wait to fire it again. It had been by my side the night before as I stared at the stars from my tiny hole, and for a second forgot about the chaos, despair, and endless violence before drifting to sleep. Each star in the black expanse was a little glint of hope during what had developed into one of the deadliest periods of the War on Terror for American troops.

My muscle memory reaction to that gunshot meant there was no time to pick up my helmet, flak jacket, or Kevlar vest—plus, it was 115 degrees and 90 percent humidity, too hot for all that garb. We wore our Kevlar, flak jacket, and helmet everywhere. Sometimes we even slept in them, even though the protective porcelain plates weighed thirty pounds, because we knew that at any minute we would have to wake up and start fighting. A shot to the helmet or Kevlar could save a Marine's life. It would hurt like hell and could cause lasting damage, but it meant there was a fighting chance of survival. I had seen Marines walk away from a shot to their gear. But in that moment I was shooting back with no protection for my head or chest, even though we were pinned down.

Our platoon was surrounded by walls of dried mud as tall as I am. If I raised my head slightly I could see what lay ahead of me: a bare Afghan landscape with nothing but sand, irrigation ditches, and poppy fields. Garmsir was made up of a few small villages dotted along the banks of the Helmand River, where farmers harvested opium on the little land that was viable. For the Taliban, it was an ideal place to fight. They knew the arid terrain like the back of their hands.

Over the mud ridge I could see a small collection of huts in the distance. The tiny mud homes on the horizon were surrounded by scraggy children's soccer balls, and connected by a network of washing lines, covered in clothes and towels that dried in seconds in the intense heat.

I scanned the windows and doorways for any target. I tracked the sniper's position instantly: he was hiding one hundred fifty feet away, behind a pile of laundry in a hut that looked like every other I had seen during my time in Afghanistan. They were simple square buildings with a hole in each wall, which sometimes had metal bars covering the windows, instead of glass. This one had a wooden roof that jutted out over where the shooter was positioned and primed.

The sniper had a clear view of our compound that would give him protection from our rifle rounds. He was taking aim at my squad and the sandbagged windows where we were squatted down. Many of my friends were in the platoon. I had spent months with them going through every emotion possible: extreme exhaustion, homesickness, violent rage, and fear. They were my world and the closest thing I had to a family in this hole in the desert. I told them how I found out I was expecting a boy, just two hours before I got on the bus bound for the airfield, to catch my flight for the deployment. I told them about my weekly calls to Bobbie on a satellite phone, where I urged her not to watch the news. The coverage of the Battle of Garmsir was like an NFL highlight reel, constantly replaying the most dramatic footage. The explosions and sound of gunfire—dramatized on widescreen TVs and amplified by surround sound systems in living rooms across the U.S.—didn't exactly put her at ease. But she knew I would constantly be thrust into dangerous situations.

With my M16 in hand, I jogged with my head down to the corner of a mud wall a few feet in front of me. I kept low, slid, and wedged myself at the bottom. I turned around and leaned on the wall with my back to the shooter. I was facing away from the target, so I was blind, but I knew roughly where he was hiding because of the tactical fire plan we had sketched out on the back of an MRE (Meal, Ready-to-Eat) packet. I really didn't like this corner: it was too exposed, and the brown mosquito netting we used to "conceal" ourselves did nothing.

Enemy marksmen like this sniper were different from the rest of the Taliban fighters. They had years of training. They were the elite, highly skilled warriors in the organization that had wreaked havoc on invading forces across Afghanistan for decades. For years they had picked off U.S. soldiers across Helmand Province, and their improved precision meant their kill count was going up. A member of this new breed had us in his crosshairs. These bastards were more capable than the average Afghan terrorist, running around waving an AK-47 above his head and spraying rounds. One shot was all this marksman would need to kill anyone stupid enough to step out into the open. One round was the difference between life and a quick but violent death, but our guys shot better.

I could already feel the unbearable heat taking its toll on my worn-out body, as I looked up from the bottom of the wall. Then more rounds started coming. The sniper had reinforcements. The pops and the ricochets were getting closer together. I could see the other Marines around me scrambling to get into position to fire back.

I wiped droplets of sweat from my forehead and got ready to slide up the wall. I pushed through the balls of my feet and straightened out my legs so my back was flush against the dirt. I grasped the rifle close to my chest and looked back toward my mouse hole and my helmet and Kevlar lying beside it.

I dropped back down so my head wasn't exposed, to consider my next move. The sweat I had wiped from my brow seconds earlier had already been replaced with new, even bigger droplets. These were heavier and filled with adrenaline. I could feel them slowly dripping down towards my eyebrows, and they turned to mud as they touched my skin. I couldn't let them get in my eyes and disrupt my line of sight, but at the same time I couldn't move. I couldn't see the sniper's eyes, but I felt them locked on me like lasers. I stabilized myself against the wall and took another deep breath. I closed my eyes for a second to clear my mind.

When I opened my eyes again, I noticed a man beside me clinging to his camera, wearing a Kevlar with "PRESS" printed on a patch on his chest. I recognized him—it was Goran Tomasevic. He was a photographer with Reuters who had embedded with our platoon a few days earlier and had been following us around, even though he didn't have a gun and couldn't defend himself. He was a nice guy, but crazy. He never shied away from the dangers that came with his job. Goran would change his lens in the middle of a hail of machine gun fire, just so a better picture could appear in newspapers or on TV screens a few days later. To him, rounds were an object that would spoil his shot, not something that could kill him.

While Marines scrambled around him and got into position, I watched as he screwed on a new, longer lens, getting ready to do his own shooting. He looked up and gave me a weird smile with very wide eyes. I didn't know whether it was nerves or excitement. All of the members of the media who followed us around without guns, just to do their jobs, were insane. They were the most vulnerable people around us, and didn't get paid nearly enough.

I couldn't pay attention to Goran. I set my sights back on the sniper's window and the pile of washed clothes he was hiding behind. I was ready to retaliate with a burst of gunfire. It would be over quickly for him if I got my shot right. He would be dead in an instant. He wouldn't feel anything. His head would violently snap back and blood would splatter all over the wall behind him. His friends would come in, scoop up his lifeless body, and carry on shooting back as if nothing had happened.

I turned my head carefully towards the top of the dirt and could see I was close to the clearing. Keeping low, I pivoted to get myself into a firing position. I pushed my right foot back behind me, spread my legs out, and started to bring my muzzle to eye-level.

I wrapped my finger around the trigger. I took one more deep breath, blinked, and went to press it back, but I didn't get that far.

A split second later my world plunged into complete darkness. At the same moment, Bobbie was in her car with one hand on the wheel and the other cradling her belly. She felt something she had never felt before. It was a jolt of sudden panic. She knew something terrible had just happened. She was convinced it wasn't a problem with her baby, but with the other man in her life on the other side of the world.

CHAPTER 2

I am a veteran in fighting the enemy, in every sense. That could be seen as an arrogant statement from an asshole Marine. But it is nothing more than a humble truth that has characterized and dominated my entire life, from the trailer parks I roamed in Ohio pretending to be my uncle fighting in Vietnam, or a kid to the suburban street in Jacksonville I now call home. I have always been guided by my own spirit and tried to be independent, but over the course of my life, I have become dependent on the people around me and have had to fight things that are out of my control: things that make me fly into a rage without any prompting, things that make me forget what I had for breakfast, things that mean I have guilt that will follow me until my funeral.

Every day there is something that reminds me I am a veteran. Since leaving the military, I have continued to become adept at dealing with all types of adversaries, because there is not one enemy, but hundreds, or thousands, and I didn't leave them behind when I returned home. They come in many forms and from all angles. They are endless, unforgiving, and ruthless, and they don't discriminate between the weak and strong, or powerful, or vulnerable. You are constantly exposed, whether you are in a desert with terrorists hiding in the hills around you or behind the trees in your backyard, while kids are playing on swing sets or neighbors are grilling ribs. I have battled many of these enemies, and I have lost more times than I can count. A few times, I only survived by mere inches. Victories are rare, and the celebration only lasts until the next fight comes along and undoubtedly gets the better of me.

When an average grunt like me tries to talk about an "enemy," many assume I am trying to describe a foreign soldier whose sole purpose is to wipe you and your fellow Marines off the face of the earth, by any means necessary. They envision men in headscarves standing in the middle of the street. To a civilian, an enemy could be defined as a terrorist who wants to strap a bomb onto himself, walk into a market, and blow hordes of men, women, and children into oblivion. It could be a member of an opposing gang wanting to gun you down in the middle of the street, or a soldier from another Army looking to take you down with a sniper shot between the eyes.

That description may be valid. But these so-called enemies aren't just in Afghanistan, Iraq, Syria, Libya, or any other battlefield around the world; they are much closer to home than you think. The enemies are among your neighbors.

Sometimes they will be obvious, but otherwise they will never manifest themselves. I'm not just talking about child molesters who are a threat to your kids when they walk home from school, serial killers who roam the streets, lone wolf gunmen who could enter a school at any time and open fire, or domestic terrorists who want to throw society into disarray.

The enemies are your wives, they are your children, they are your friends, they are your family, your bartenders, your garbage men, PTA members; they are the strangers you pass in the street. Their threat isn't obvious and certainly isn't visible. It is hidden in a place you may never be able to find. They may not be carrying guns or knives, but they still pose a danger. That is because your main enemy is you.

I have recurring dreams of the sounds of explosions, whether they are in a desert in South West Asia or playing on repeat in your head, from what should be the comfort of your bedroom. Then I see the faces of the Marines for whose deaths I feel responsible. The enemy isn't just the Taliban, Al Qaeda, or the Islamic State; it isn't terrorists with their pashmina scarves waving AK-47s above their heads, walking into markets with suicide vests packed with nails or ball-bearings. The enemy is the government that has abandoned those it's supposed to be looking after—not providing the best care for servicemen and women who almost died fighting for its people. The enemy is the cocktail of eighteen drugs you have been prescribed that could kill you when taken together; the constant memory loss; the violent outbursts you can't control; and the thoughts that you could just end it all with two bottles of tequila, a shot glass, and a note to your long-suffering wife.

There are many times I was inches from giving up, because I couldn't deal with it anymore. Nearly every time, the problems were with me. I couldn't deal with the man I had become: a distant father to my son and an absent husband to my wife. The flashbacks come at random. They are sparked by a sound no one else can hear, or something no one else can see. Some of the memories are good, but most are bad. They come back every time I see those photos taken by Goran Tomasevic of my close call with the Taliban sniper round, the dirt exploding in front of my face, and me collapsing to the ground in a hail of gunfire. The world goes black, or I am back lying on a stretcher. I remember the horror of the next few hours. The images were broadcast around the world, and made headlines at a time when millions of Americans were questioning why we were even fighting in Afghanistan in the first place. They were shared to show the bravery of every single person fighting overseas for the U.S. after 9/11, during the hunt for terrorists around the world, but some would see it as a moment of utter stupidity. People don't understand why a man would take on the enemy wearing just a T-shirt and pants. It is simply a reality of the unpredictable nature of living on a battlefield.

These photos would make for a great poster on any thirteen-year-old boy's wall, and even resulted in me being in a video game. They are dramatic and exciting to the average person, but they set my life on a course of destruction that I couldn't avoid. No one really knows the idiot in the photograph who almost died and left his pregnant wife a widow. I was the dumbass who picked up his rifle, but left his helmet and Kevlar in the sand. Now, when I open news stories or watch a TV show about the war, often photos of me will come up. They are used constantly to depict the violence in Afghanistan, and are illustrations for articles in the endless debate about America's longest war that has cost the U.S. roughly one trillion dollars over twenty years—more than the Apollo moon landing, the Manhattan Project, and the Marshall Plan. Some of the interpreters I worked with, who risked their lives for the U.S., were left behind when our troops finally left. 2,372 American military members, including my friends, were killed in the country. Countless more have been lost since, and more will die in years to come.

Those photos show me when I was just inches from death, and they will forever define me in the public eye, wherever I go and for as long as I live—not the photos of me with a tear in my eye when I got the Purple Heart in 2016, not the hours spent taking on the Taliban, not the Marines around me who sacrificed their lives and became my family.

In 2010, I returned from my final tour with the Marines earlier than expected. There were still thousands of U.S. troops fighting in Afghanistan, and it didn't seem like they would be leaving any time soon. They still haven't. Much like Vietnam, it was hard to tell what progress—if any—was being made. The U.S. had gotten itself into a war that had gone on far longer than anyone had hoped for, and it ended in disaster, with the very people we tried to eradicate back in power.

I read reports that the Pentagon had lied about progress in the war to save the embarrassment of the stalled headway. Generals lied and threw thousands of young Marines to the dogs. While they were sitting in their ivory towers choosing drone targets, we were sweating in the sand and exposed to the vicious, American-hating Taliban. We were battling every day in dirty clothes and surviving on terrible military-issued food, for an endgame that wasn't even on the horizon.

Not much has changed. What I see never changes. It replays over and over again, in between all of the other bad memories I have tried to store away, so the people close to me don't have to share the pain: every close encounter, every gunfight, every friend I have lost, every nighttime patrol. I am no longer in one of the hottest places on earth, surrounded by psychopathic suicide bombers and ruthless jihadi fighters with a purpose many will never understand. I am no longer faced with gun battles every six hours, or the prospect of laying down my head to sleep every night in a hole in the dirt, listening to more gun battles going on just a few feet away.

Now, I am in my bedroom in Jacksonville with my wife beside me. Instead of endless stretches of barren land and poppy fields, I see well-manicured grass on front lawns and driveways with mid-range sedans that symbolize quiet suburban life. My neighbors will walk past, wave to me and shout "good morning" like everything is normal. It should be a welcome change from Afghanistan. But under the surface the signs of my war are still there and tangled up in my everyday routine. I can't escape, and yet I would give anything to be back on the front lines leading my squad.

Simple everyday items can spark flashbacks. Trash reminds me of one of the most common tactics used by terrorist combatants: IEDs hidden in garbage.

I have to walk around our neighborhood and see piles of trash dotted around. I could be outside with a cigarette or playing with my son. The trash is all around me. When I drive to work or head to the mall, I see trash everywhere. I'm not scared it will blow up in my face, but it takes my mind back to Helmand Province. I tell myself that I am being ridiculous, but it is impossible to simply set my experiences from the war aside. It's more than the garbage I pass—it's also people in a grocery store when I get disorientated or frustrated in the produce aisle. The anger that overwhelms me in civilian life was an invaluable tool to me when taking on the Taliban. These normal aspects of civilian life are things I have had to try to adapt to since I returned from the war. Bobbie went through hell while I was away; now she is going through hell at home with my nightmares, memory loss, anger, and times where I go deep into the darkest places of my mind.

I can walk around with a smile on my face and laugh at any joke, no matter how bad it might be. I am able to put on a brave positive face and hide the pain most of the time. But in reality, I am living in darkness, like the darkness I fell into when the sniper round hit the bank just a few inches from my head.

I can hear the gunshots and explosions at night, during the day, while I am playing with my son, while I am hanging out with my family, and while I am getting groceries at Walmart. It is never-ending. It is on repeat, and I can't switch it off no matter how hard I try. No matter how much I drink, how much cannabis I smoke, or how many prescribed pills I take, I constantly feel like I flew back from my final tour and was just dropped back into another warzone with no protection around me. What should be quiet nights at home have turned into Bobbie dealing with my violent and erratic outbursts that often come from nowhere.

I am by no means a good person. I am angry, violent, and have little to no patience. I swear too much, and sometimes go internal for months at a time, not talking to anyone. These problems sometimes turn to suicidal thoughts. I ask myself: *What is the point of carrying on if I am going to go through this hell every day? Do I want my son growing up in a house with me tucking him into bed at night? Should I do something to myself before I do something to someone else?*

I have stacked sweaters neatly in the fridge and put my cigarettes in milk jugs. I had absolutely no idea how they got there, and I couldn't find a reason why I put them there. I normally can't explain my actions. I have needed help for years, and I still need it. Normally, the only person there for me is my wife. My four-foot-eleven, 125-pound line of defense is one of the only things stopping me from doing something very dangerous and potentially hurting someone. I should have been given, and still should be getting, constant care from the government I risked my life for. But as soon as I got back from the war, I was simply cast aside by a tainted bureaucratic system—the Department of Veterans Affairs (known as the VA). It has become a government agency notorious for scandal. Dealing with these public issues and its poor image means it has often been distracted from its primary task: looking after servicemen and women when they return home.

Many former service members have had very different experiences from me with what has become one of the most controversial taxpayer-funded entities in the United States. Mine has been very mixed. There have been some positives, including the nurses who look after you before appointments, or are there when you have an emergency. They are often the first line of defense, and the best one at that. Beyond them is utter confusion.

Thousands, maybe millions, of people have seen me just inches from death, and in one of the most intimate moments anyone could experience. But only my family, friends, doctors, nurses, and a few Marines know the whole story. I have only recently been able to build up the courage to tell my close family and friends what I went through in Helmand Province, and describe what people didn't read in the news stories or watch on TV news.

Back in 2015, Wills Robinson—a journalist with Daily-Mail.com and the co-author of this book—wrote to me asking if he could interview me for an article on me and my life, since those photos were taken. It was the first time details about my life had ever been published. It helped me to open up, and I have been more forthcoming ever since, and my spotty memory has recalled a clearer picture of what happened. At first, I wanted to ignore Wills' emails, because I didn't like the idea of sharing my journey with someone who hadn't been through the same things I have. They just don't understand. I didn't want to complain about my circumstances, because there are veterans whose situations are far more terrible than I could comprehend. I spoke to Bobbie and my sister Kristan—my sounding boards when I needed to talk something through—and they said the story of what happened in Afghanistan, and my life when I came home, needed to be told, because thousands of others have had similar experiences. They have been through the hell that is Helmand Province: the brutal fire-fights, the evil of the Taliban, the IED blasts; they know what it is like to feel responsible for your friends' deaths.

In the decade since I returned home from a military hospital in Germany, I have been battling with myself over whether to share my journey with the world. I detest being portrayed as a hero and always get uncomfortable when someone thanks me for my service, but I want to help people like me. If I wanted to be compared to the likes of G.I. Joe or *American Sniper* Chris Kyle, or turn myself into a warrior straight from a Tom Clancy novel, then I would have come forward years ago. I read all the articles and books from the officers and operators, and struggled to find many from the perspective of infantrymen who spent weeks living in dirt away from air-conditioned base offices and faced the toughest obstacles when they returned home to American soil. Like the men I fought with, they were just grunts who wanted to protect their country and find and kill whoever was responsible for 9/11. I loved being a Marine, and was very good at my job when I was deployed, and sometimes I ask myself what would have happened if my career hadn't been brought to an abrupt end. The contents of this book contain everything I can recall to the best of my abilities. I hope that my story serves as a way to remind people that we may be seen as heroes when we return home, but we don't feel that way and sometimes are certainly not treated that way. I loved protecting and serving my country, and I wish I could go back overseas and do my job all over again, but what happened meant that was simply not possible.

CHAPTER 3

I showed up in the classroom, got behind my desk in front of the whiteboard, and looked at my watch. I was fifteen minutes early.

I hate being late. It might be due to the military discipline instilled in me since I arrived at boot camp in 2000, and from being on time to pointless formations where young Marines would stand in rectangles for hours on end. Presently, I looked from wall to wall to see my students were relaxed and mingling like it was a normal day. They were talking to each other, cracking jokes and laughing, and it brought a smile to my face, because I knew that for many of them, my class on transitioning from service to civilian life was far from easy. *Was I doing a good job for them? Was I teaching them the right things?* These thoughts were always lingering at the back of my mind, because I was responsible for making sure they had the best chance to not only survive, but thrive, in the world outside the military.

I was working as an instructor at the Veterans Benefits Administration, because I still hadn't been given the medical retirement Bobbie had spent years fighting for, and the benefits for my three traumatic brain injuries only covered a small amount of our expenses.

I use the word "students" in the loosest sense. They weren't ignorant thirteen-year-old schoolchildren waiting to go home and trying to make a teacher's life hell whenever possible. I was not teaching them algebra, making them memorize the periodic table, or asking them to write essays on *The Great Gatsby* and *Catcher in the Rye*. They weren't dissecting frogs or learning how to ask for an ice cream in Spanish. My class didn't have finals at the end of the semester, and I didn't give them detention if they acted up or talked out of turn. No, they certainly weren't children, and they had experienced far more trauma and horror in life than many people in a normal classroom ever had or would.

They had all been to, fought on, and then returned home from the front lines. They had traveled to different corners of the globe to fight for their country. Many of them had been overseas, seen and experienced the same things I had, and were now trying to figure out what was next. My job was to try to help them back to some sort of normalcy. It was a struggle for all of them, but it was a struggle I am very familiar with.

Most of them—thankfully—had all of their limbs intact and were excited to get on with their lives. But some had to pull themselves through the classroom door in wheelchairs, or hobble on crutches. Others had patches over their eyes, while a couple sitting at the back had one arm each in a sling. A pair on the right side of the room had missing arms. If you put a group of fifty or so wounded veterans in the same room anywhere in America, the dynamic would be pretty much the same. I knew they were fortunate to be there at all because I knew too many that weren't.

All of them had one thing in common: their battle-hardened faces staring at a future of uncertainty with a hint of hope. I felt like I could see straight through their beards and tattoos into their souls that had been injured beyond repair. The swelling may go down and the scars may fade, but the wounds never disappear.

Even though they had been through hell, they knew the immediate threat was establishing a plan for what to do next. Not only did they have to recover from the mental or physical injuries they had suffered in poppy fields or deserts thousands of miles from home, they had to start life over again. They had to get a job, save what little they had of their military salary, and try to find a place to live. I didn't want them to end up living in their cars or on a sidewalk.

Like me, they didn't have the protection of a uniform anymore. They couldn't walk into a mess hall and get three square meals a day. The food in the Marines wasn't great, but it was better than being homeless and not knowing where your next meal was coming from.

For some it is an easy transition, while for others it may seem an impossible task, especially with no help. At least I had Bobbie there to stop me going adrift, and Ethan to motivate me to become a better father. For some of these students taking classes in the Veterans Benefits Administration, I was one of the only options they had in their post-service life. Many of them, like me, had joined the Marines straight out of high school after 9/11. Boot camp was the first time they had lived away from their parents. For some of them, like me, it was the first time they had traveled outside the U.S. The farthest I had traveled without my family was from Ohio to a church camp in Washington State.

In the worst instances, they might use the little money they had to buy drugs to try to dull the pain. What they knew before the war was playing football on a Friday night in front of their town, drinking beers with friends, playing video games in the basement when they were supposed to be doing homework, and trying to get a girl in class to like them. Now, some were thinking about going to college, while others were simply trying to pass the SATs.

After five years of teaching, I was a novice and still learning how to get my message across. I shared stories—some funny and some horrific—to try to get them to relate to me.

"Gentleman, it's time to learn from the master. Get ready for eight hours of PowerPoint slides," I shouted, with a small smile on my face. They quickly stopped their chitchat and fell quiet. They still had the sense of discipline and order that had been drilled into them from the first day they enlisted. It's something that is instilled in Marines their whole life, and is an attribute difficult to get rid of.

They pulled out notepads from their backpacks. Some had to use computers because they had lost their writing hand. I had to produce a sheet with all my lecture points for those who couldn't concentrate for the whole session, so they could reread it when they got home. (Brain injuries normally result in severe problems with retaining information.)

I tried to be as entertaining as I could be when giving my lessons. Most of my jokes fell flat, but some lifted these guys' spirits and made them laugh like they would at a bar over a beer. As I drove to class, I would rehearse my lines while Ethan sat in the back with a blank stare.

"Today, guys, we are talking about resumes," I told the class once they had settled down. "Many of you will have never thought about them, because most of you have only had one job: fighting and cleaning crusty underwear. Some of you may have actually learned a job skill at your MOS school, other than shooting things and blowing shit up. But this is crucial, and I will try my best to make sure you don't end up living in a van down by the river." I heard some quiet chuckles across the room from those who knew the line from Chris Farley's infamous 1993 *Saturday Night Live* sketch. "You only need to be able to write your name to sign up for the war. But this is different. You need to sell yourself. Just putting 'Grunt' in your 'work experience' section, followed by your summer flipping burgers at Wendy's or mowing your neighbor's lawn, won't really work when you are trying to become an investment banker with a Ferrari in the driveway, if you know what I mean."

They all burst out laughing and one even shouted "Oorah" while banging his fist on the desk in front of him. I looked around the classroom and laughed a little to myself, but I noticed one of the men at the end of one of the rows didn't even raise a smile, and barely flinched. He was alone and seemed like he was trapped in his own thoughts.

He was just staring down at the floor with a glum, emotionless expression on his face. Maybe he hadn't heard what I'd said. Some of the men had problems hearing, and others would zone out easily as soon as another thought crept into their head. I tried my best to accommodate everyone and make sure I gave them my full attention during classes.

When the class stopped high-fiving and settled down again, I turned around to the screen to start my presentation. It wasn't much more than a PowerPoint presentation I had to memorize, listing veteran benefits and classes, plus a few bullet points I had scribbled in my instructor's guide the night before, with the help of Bobbie and a couple of beers.

The reality was that if I ever wrote a resume, Bobbie would proofread it. I would give her a version, she would completely rewrite it, and then she would give it back to me. She'd translate everything I wrote into terms a non-military employer would understand and have to fix the dates. I couldn't trust myself to present my background in a resume; the issues with my brain messed with my perceptions of time. Something I thought had happened a few months prior could have actually been years before, and I would forget events that had happened a few days earlier.

I turned back to the class and my eyes turned to the guy who had been bowing his head, and I saw his hand was raised. He still looked empty of emotion, but he was looking right at me. It looked like a thought had finally popped into his head. I nodded in his direction to give him permission to speak, and the rest of the class gave him their silence.

"Sir," he said, very quietly. I hated when these guys called me "Sir." We weren't in the service anymore and I was never a "Sir". I wanted them to treat me as a friend and an equal; I wasn't there to lead their patrol or send them out to clear a building that could be full of explosives.

I grinned and said to him: "Man, come on, it's Bill. I'm not paid to be an asshole. We aren't *in* anymore. We are all equals here. Aside from the fact that I am far better looking than your ugly ass." There was another laugh that showed the guys were still in good spirits. The glum Marines's mouth raised at the sides with a hint of a smile, and I was hoping he could open up if he were a bit more relaxed.

"Sorry, Bill," he said back. "I just wanted to ask you something before we started the class today. I was reading about the VA last night. I typed the letters into Google and an article came up from a Florida news website. I clicked on it and just saw a picture of a hospital with a pretty disturbing headline about a veteran from Tampa. I hated it and had to stop for a second and compose myself. I didn't think something like it was possible. You know what the news media is like, they pick out the negatives, so I try to take everything they say or write with a pinch of salt. But this was pretty bad. In fact, it was depressing as hell."

Most of these guys were struggling with the VA, just like I was. It was in the early stages of setting up a healthcare program, based on the conditions servicemen had picked up during their service that could require round-the-clock care or constant therapy for psychological problems. I was getting caught up in the same bureaucracy they were, being bounced between doctors and getting a hoard of antipsychotic medication to numb the pain and ease the relentless trauma. My aim was to keep my students as positive as I could about what they could expect in their care, when the reality was slightly different.

The Marine continued. "An elderly Army vet who must have been in his seventies or eighties died in the shower at this hospital," he said. "I think he served in Korea. I can't remember off the top of my head. He must have slipped or fallen over and couldn't get back up off the ground. I found it weird that there wasn't a rail he could use. Maybe he couldn't pull himself up. But he just lay there, with the shower water still running over his body. The nurses left his body there for nine hours. He died alone and his body was left to shrivel. There weren't many details, other than an investigation had been launched. They didn't say whether he had been burned, but he would have been in a very bad shape.

"The poor man could have survived if the medical staff had gotten to him faster. All they needed to do was check up on him to see if he was okay, so why didn't they come into his room for nine hours? He was frail, and a nurse couldn't have been more than ten feet away from him at any time. It's a horrible way to die, considering the sacrifices this guy made for our country. He left this world in the most undignified way, and it wasn't his fault."

The tone in his voice grew more scared, the more he spoke. All of the men were looking at him, and they were terrified too. "What if I needed to go to this hospital?" the Marine went on. "What if I wanted a shower and I slipped and fell? Is it really too much to ask for someone to help me up? Is it too much for someone to come in and check on me, if I can't move myself? If I can't do anything for myself? What if I don't have any family, or friends, to help me?

"Is this our reality now, Bill? Is this the way we are going to be treated until we die, however long we may have left to live? I have been on tours. I have been shot at more times than I can count, and my friends have died. All this while the people living around us question why America is fighting the war. The least I can expect is a basic level of care from the government I almost died for. The least I deserve is human decency."

The truth was I had read the same horrifying, disgusting report. It made me sick to the stomach thinking someone like me had been left on the ground, in their own filth, to die. The nurses must have been at their station, just on the other side of the door. I tried to imagine what would have been going through the man's mind at that time, and whether I would go through the same thing. It was the kind of article I had gotten used to reading about the VA.

During the Revolutionary War, Congress encouraged soldiers to keep fighting the British by promising they would be paid when they returned from the front lines. It was a small amount of compensation to avoid mass desertions, and the first pension program controlled by the federal government.

The payments were left up to the states—or rather, the thirteen colonies that existed at the time—but hardly any of the troops got their money when they got home, even though they helped form the country we live in today. It paved the way for more generous pension and aid programs in the military, but over the next two hundred years, there was little improvement in care for ex-servicemen and women.

Warren Harding—probably the most hated and corrupt president in the history of the United States—appointed his longtime friend and crony Charles Forbes as head of the newly formed Veterans Bureau in 1921—the government department that would eventually turn into the Department of Veterans Affairs. Forbes—with the help of staff like Charles Cramer, an official in his department—was tasked with providing medical care for the millions of ex-servicemen and women who survived the First World War. More than 116,000 American men fought in the trenches in some of the most horrific conditions seen in modern warfare and came home with shell shock, or shrapnel embedded in their bodies. They needed all the help they could get, especially with the limits of medicine at the time. Instead, Forbes stole and embezzled more than $200 million from the government set aside for veterans' hospitals. He was sentenced to two years in prison; Charles Cramer committed suicide.

As a bookworm and history nerd since elementary school, this scandal fascinated me. The battles and operations are often what is most reported and celebrated in military history. Society and the economy are mostly taken care of in the aftermath, but the soldiers who were on the frontline—and are now back picking up the pieces—get overlooked. I didn't want to tell the guys in front of me that this was the reality they now faced. It would have been easy to say all of the problems faced by veterans were set firmly in the past, but it would have been a blatant lie.

I remember watching a press conference with former President Donald Trump's then VA Secretary David Shulkin. He said veterans were driving onto the grounds of VA hospitals or medical facilities and killing themselves. Some would shoot themselves, others would set themselves on fire, all in a desperate act to draw attention to the failure in care they were experiencing.

As a Marine, I was too familiar with suicide, from my friends choosing to end their lives when they finished deployments, to my time as a Suicide Prevention Trainer, or one of my many brushes of death that came when I decided drinking two bottles of tequila as fast as I could would be an appropriate way to die. But I didn't want to give them a bleak outlook, so I told them my story in a way I thought would give them hope. They all looked up to me because they had seen the series of photos of me that had been published over and over again, and which constantly reminded me of my many ups and downs.

My smiles as their teacher were all for show, because the reality was I was suffering from random flashbacks, outbursts of pure anger, memory loss, and traumatic brain injuries that caused sleepwalking and meant I couldn't run more than three hundred yards without falling sick or losing my balance. I woke up in the middle of the night screaming because I could hear the sound of gunfire, or I would get lost in Walmart while smelling grenade smoke that wasn't there. I wanted them to know I kept falling into an abyss, fearing I would never make it back out, and I was still begging the VA to let me regularly see a psychiatrist and a head specialist.

CHAPTER 4

By just eight years of age, I had already developed survival instincts and experienced the isolation I needed to become a grunt. I grew up in the ass-end of nowhere, in a trailer park between the Ohio cities of Wooster and Mansfield, about sixty miles south of Cleveland. You would only hear about either city in the news if there was a mass shooting, or a politician flew in to hold a rally. There was nothing but factories, where most of my family worked at some point in their lives, bordered by miles of farmland and cornfields. Planes flying over would see vast stretches of land and the chimneys of the paper and steel mills. It was true Rust Belt America; most of the families were working class, living paycheck to paycheck, and struggling to get food on the table.

My parents split up when I was two. I don't remember what happened, so I had to rely on my sister Kristan, who was two years older than me, to explain how our home was suddenly ripped apart. To this day, I firmly believe it is one of the events that helped shape the fighter I became.

Our parents got joint custody so we would spend the week with my mom in her trailer and the weekend with my dad in his.

My mom worked at the paper factory in Wooster, while my dad spent his days at the steel mill. Their jobs had them away from home most of the day and when they got back they were too exhausted to play with us. But they got food on the table and a roof over our heads, and that's all that mattered when every day was a struggle. Kristan was the best person to have at my side. We were inseparable as we fended for ourselves in the desolate rural environment where we spent the bulk of our childhood. We formed an unbreakable bond and helped each other climb over every obstacle, because we were in it together and had to mature very quickly.

My dad suffered the tragic combination of working his ass off only for the factory to shut down and be moved out of state or overseas. He bounced between jobs and often didn't have a paycheck. On the weekends, he would take us to the Orrville Moose Lodge or the American Legion where he'd let us play anything we wanted on the jukebox. My sister and I played pool for hours and we were in heaven.

We spent a lot of time at our step grandma's house, where I first learned to shoot, and picked up skills like gardening and cooking. She would take me out to the back of the house, give me her rifle, and teach me the basics of marksmanship. Her favorite targets were any animals that tried to get into her garden. Most often it was groundhogs, but she was known to kill the occasional brave deer with a headshot from seventy-five yards.

My mom moved on from my dad and married my step-father Danny, a kind and patient man who worked at the same factory as her and lived a few trailers up from us. He was a cannoneer in the Army, and I grew to like him pretty quickly, even though he had entered our lives in the middle of utter chaos. He only raised his voice at me a handful of times when I was a kid, and he was good to me.

Kristan and I would barely see our mom and stepdad during the week. They would leave for their shift first thing in the morning before we got up, and get home late in the evening. She put food on the table while working grueling hours, but we barely had any money left over for other survival.

When my mom and stepdad left for work, our step-grandma—as we called her—would be forced to watch us during the day. She would lock us out of the trailer, because she firmly believed children should spend as much time outside as possible. She didn't care what we would get up to until it was time to return, have a shower, and eat dinner. This helped develop my love of nature and exploration, and instilled in me the fundamentals of bushcraft and navigation.

Kristan and I would ride our bikes everywhere we could, and explore the depths of the woods and the cornfields. We would walk for miles on end until we couldn't bear another step, and every time we returned home our clothes were covered in filth. We would dig around the mud looking for nothing in particular, track animals, build tree houses out of wood scraps, and climb onto branches so we could swing on them without a care in the world. Kristan and I were always playing games where I could imagine myself in battle by hiding in the undergrowth and chasing her down from every flank. I would put on Danny's old Army cammies and gear and imagine I was on patrol trying to track bad guys, with my sister playing the part of the enemy and ambushing me. There was no end to the trouble we could get into.

We would build forts out of fallen branches and twigs. I would take my stepdad's army uniform and put it on, and we would run around with toy guns pretending we were in the middle of a battlefield thousands of miles away. I would lie down in the mud and crawl towards my enemy target with streaks of dirt under my eyes, and would take cover behind trees for hours, getting ready for my imaginary ambush. The Marine in me was already growing in my blood and bones, and without knowing it I was already on a path in life.

I was surrounded by military men growing up, and knew that one day I would end up serving, after hearing stories about the honor of serving their country. Bees had served in the military for generations—starting with the Revolutionary War and leading up to my grandfather who was in World War II, and my uncle in Vietnam—and when I went into the woods I pretended to be them. At six years old, I was already obsessed with military movies, and would piss off my sister by playing the 1980s film *Tank* on repeat during the little time we had to sit and watch TV, and would act out the plot from *Predator* in one of our many imaginary scenarios in the woods.

The issue with being left alone for so long—with only my sister to supervise—was that I was getting into trouble. I wasn't an evil child, and I never had any real criminal intentions, but my inquisitiveness got the better of me and I started breaking into other trailers. I had to do anything to stop myself from getting bored, and for a smart kid, it was the dumbest decision I could have made. I would never take anything valuable. All I would do was pop in and rummage around and then run back out. It seemed like a foolproof plan and was a hell of a lot of fun, until I was caught trying to get into a trailer in the park where we were living. The owners were furious and marched me over to my mom's trailer by the scruff of my shirt.

I felt lucky they had decided against calling the cops. But how would my mom punish me? Would she ground me and have my step-grandma lock me out of the house again, so I could carry on running riot around the neighborhood? It turned out that my mom had had enough with my endless antics while she was at work trying to provide for us, and she decided it was time to truly teach me a lesson by throwing me into the back seat of her car, and driving me to the police station. I was terrified and crying my eyes out. I'd had encounters with cops, and run away from officers a few times into the woods before, but this time I would be in the same building as the sheriff and the jail. I stepped onto the sidewalk outside the local police headquarters, shaking with nerves from head to toe, and with my hands in my pockets. My mom approached the front desk and the officer on duty and told him what I had done. He was wearing a broad-brimmed hat that I had seen on cowboys in films and books, and the silver sheriff's badge stared at me menacingly from his chest. I was in the presence of serious authority, and I was petrified.

"I should arrest you. I could do that," he said. He looked at my mom with a smirk and reached down and touched the top of his handcuffs, while my heart started pounding faster. He then grabbed me by the arm and dragged me along a corridor lined by officers at their desks in uniform, doing paperwork and making phone calls. As I reached the end of the hallway towards the back of the police station, I saw a concrete slab with a head pillow at one end and a metal toilet bowl at the other. The sheriff pulled me inside, sat me on the bed, and said to me: "Stay there." Then I saw the door lined with metal bars and started to panic. He took a huge metal ring of what seemed like a hundred keys from his pocket and jangled them in front of my face, and then I watched as he closed the door shut with a bang and locked it. I stayed there sobbing with my knees together and my head in my hands for what seemed like hours—when it had only been a few minutes—and waited until he let me out. He knew I wouldn't be breaking into trailers in the near future.

In third grade I was a nightmare for my teachers. I was the hyper kid who would always sit at the front of the class, constantly fidget in my seat, and ask questions whenever I wasn't supposed to. I drove the staff teachers crazy and it got to be too much for them, so they sent me to a doctor for a series of tests. Little did I know these medical exams would come back to haunt me. For months I was sent to the hospital for a series of appointments where I would sit in a room for two hours, with wires attached to my head, while they monitored me. This went on for months before I was finally diagnosed with ADHD.

Despite the diagnosis and getting into trouble at home, at school I was building up a sense of discipline and structure. I read like no one else my age and would dive into the biggest books I could get my hands on, to take to the cornfields or my dad's trailer to keep myself occupied. Books were where I got a lot of my ideas for our adventures and where I learned everything about my surroundings. When I was in elementary school, I finished Charles Dickens' *A Tale of Two Cities*, and by the time I was ten I was enjoying Anne Rice novels. I couldn't put them down, and the few friends I had thought I was the purest nerd they would ever encounter. We attended Northwestern, a small school with a graduating class of less than seventy. Anonymity was never really an option; everyone knew each other and had since kindergarten. I was a tiny kid at barely five feet tall, and I didn't make it to ninety-five pounds until I graduated from high school. I made it onto the wrestling team as a scrappy fighter, where I could use my small size to my advantage, but I was still extremely timid and needed my sister to step in whenever I was being picked on. The volatile temper that carried through my adult life started when I was a kid, and I was never one to stand down. Kristan was a lot bigger than me, and if I ever got into a fight on the playground, she would run in and beat the crap out of anyone who tried to take me on. It got to a point where none of the other kids would pick on me because they were so scared of her, even though they knew they could beat me to a pulp if they wanted to. She had been watching over me since we were in diapers, and she never stopped looking after me.

One of the ways I took out my frustration with everything going on around me was the drums. I played with the same obsession as a cocaine addict. My school life revolved around music. I signed up for every band I could and would carry my bass drum around with me like a rifle. I had the reputation of a band geek and bookworm, but felt authority strolling the corridors with my drum wrapped around my shoulders. I felt music was my calling and thought that it would be my way into the Marines, since the U.S. wasn't involved in any major overseas combat at the time. The First Gulf War had ended a few years earlier, and there were only a few skirmishes in Somalia. I thought that joining the music regiments would be the way forward, and that I could carry on my passion for music while serving my country—but God had other ideas for me.

Even though we were banished from our step-grandma's trailer most of the time, Kristan and I did everything we could to get away from the trailer park. We went to church two or three times a week, to get away from the toxic environment that was a constant reminder of our helter-skelter upbringing. I didn't get too involved in the social network of the church until high school, when I realized I wasn't Mr. Popular, and began to see the church as a chance to meet more people.

It led to Kristan's and my first trip away without our parents, on a mission trip to Washington State when I was a freshman in high school. It was a huge deal for my sister and me because we had virtually no money, but we had saved up pocket money for this trip by working part-time in a restaurant, where my sister would waitress and I would work in the kitchen. It was the farthest we had ever been away from home, and a far cry from our trips to Pennsylvania to visit family once a year, where we would sleep on the floor or couches.

I had only read about and seen photos of the Pacific Ocean, but never could have imagined how vast and beautiful it would look up close. Kristan and I drove to the coast during a break from knocking on doors spreading the word of God, and saw the waves crashing onto the beach. We were in awe and just sat in the car in silence for minutes staring out towards the horizon. Finally we got out, walked down towards the sand, and took off our shoes to let the salt water wash over our feet. The water coming down from the Arctic was freezing, but we didn't move. We wedged our feet further into the sand, and listened to the movement of the water and the seagulls flying above calling to each other. As I gazed at the Pacific Ocean, I imagined all the places I could go and all the other oceans I could visit around the world, after being stuck in Ohio my entire childhood. When I was old enough, I was going to get the freedom I needed to do what I had always wanted to: be a Marine. In less than two years—at just seventeen, and before the end of high school—I would be signing up to serve my country.

The summer before my senior year of high school, I went to a recruitment office for every branch of the military to weigh my options. I had always been passionate about the mystique and the history of the Marines, but I needed to be sure I had made the right decision. The Navy told me I could work in a nuclear reactor on a ship, but that wasn't for me. The Air Force tried to wow me with the work of electronic warfare information specialists, but I didn't want to do that. The Army came the closest to persuading me, and kept me in their office for the longest time by telling me I could become a Ranger: the elite unit given the most intense training in the Army, and always battle-ready so that they could go into a warzone before the rest of the infantry. But when I walked into the door of the Marine recruitment office, a sergeant was hanging from the doorway doing chin-ups. He was barely breaking a sweat, and breathing easily as he bent his elbows and pushed his head above the bar. He heard me come in and turned his neck so he could see me out of the corner of his eye, then let out a sigh. He dropped to the floor with a thud and, without looking at me, raised his hand and waved his fingers to tell me to follow him.

I took a chair on the other side of his desk, and for the next two hours he told me I would be insane to choose to wear the Marine uniform. He warned me I needed to think long and hard about what I was doing, and if I just wanted to gain a new skill or get free college tuition or free healthcare, I should leave and never come back. He said I would suffer the worst physical and mental pain imaginable. He said that I would go to places so cold you would have to hold a plastic water bottle against your skin to stop it from freezing, and places so hot the same bottle would melt in your hands and the water would boil. I would go for months without showering, with my underwear so dirty it would start rotting, and socks so crusty they would stand upright on their own, and I would sit in a dark cave in a country thousands of miles away, or in a town I had never heard of, where the population wanted to kill you. But, he said, I would be closer than anyone to the enemies of the United States. I would be able to take down the most evil bastards on the planet—those who didn't just deserve death, but required it. I would be able to channel the purest patriotism into one of the toughest jobs on the planet. Growing up, I knew there were bad guys that needed to be killed to keep us safe, and I was committed to make a change, so I was sold.

Because I was only seventeen and joining up before graduation, I had to get permission from my parents. My dad gave me his full support, but my mom wasn't happy, and really wanted me to follow in her footsteps and work in one of the factories. There was no way I was going to take a job that had turned my parents into shells of themselves, and turn my back on a career I had spent my childhood dreaming of. After endless hours of my begging and almost throwing tantrums, my mom gave in and signed the papers to make her son a grunt.

Over the next months, I started physically preparing myself for boot camp by working out and riding my bike every day for twenty minutes, through the dirt lanes and grass around the trailer park, and into downtown Wooster. My mind was laser focused. The Marines was all I could think about while I studied, went to band practice, and hung out with friends. I graduated from Northwestern in June 2000, and cemented my place in the Marines with my GED. Eleven days later, carrying only the tiny backpack I was permitted to bring with me, I took the bus with a group of boys my age to Parris Island depot for new recruits in South Carolina, stupidly believing that a childhood spent shooting with my step-grandma in her backyard, roaming the fields around Ohio with my sister, and my chaotic childhood would make me the perfect cadet.

The bus rolled up to the depot in the middle of the night, some of the boys looking excited and others more terrified than I could possibly imagine. I was ready for the madness and the stress the drill instructors would throw my way for the next four weeks, as they transformed me from a civilian into a warrior. The drill instructors in their wide-brimmed hats screamed at us to get off the bus and marched us into a parking lot, while the rest of the camp was sleeping. We were ordered to stand on pairs of yellow painted footprints, which symbolized the starting point of our Marine journey, and a reminder that thousands of men who joined before us had stood in the same spot.

They sat me down in a barber's chair and gave me the Marine high-and-tight haircut that would become my signature look for the next decade. Then I picked up my uniform and sneakers. I was ready for the physical side of training, but certainly not the psychological. No matter who you are, or where you are from, you are treated like a slab of beef being turned into a steak. The instructors are intimidating to the point of being downright psychotic, and spend every hour trying to wear you down and break you apart. People ask whether boot camp is the same as in the 1987 movie *Full Metal Jacket*, in which every recruit is belittled with tirades of swearing and insults that would make even the toughest man squirm. In reality, drill sergeants don't curse; instead, they find the most articulate ways to make you feel as small as possible. I came to know the main enforcer, also known as the "kill hat," very well. While the other instructors teach you the basics and history of the Marine Corps, the kill hat's sole job is to make you suffer to the point where you give up, pack your bags, and head back to whatever ass-end hometown you came from. He would play mind games, and make the platoon spend nine hours cleaning the squad bay with toothbrushes until it was spotless. The kill hat would then walk in, flip the entire room back onto the floor in huge piles because he found a rifle out of place, and tell us we had fifteen minutes to clear it up.

I breezed through most of the classroom sessions because I was a history buff and had no problems passing the written tests, but one of my biggest challenges were the hikes. I was so short I had to travel twice the distance of everyone around me, and with the huge backpacks and weapons weighing me down. It was grueling until I settled into the intense workouts and physical exercise of boot camp, and got in better shape. When I finished school, I was wrestling at 119 pounds; I was now 160 pounds of almost pure muscle and no body fat.

The whole experience was a test in mental endurance. You were knocked down and ridiculed at every opportunity, and you also had a responsibility to the rest of your unit. You were in it together, and if one recruit slipped up, then the rest of you would be punished. Boot camp removes every sense of individuality you have, and words like "I" or "me" are banned. You may think it was "every man for himself" in an environment where everyone is being tested to their limits and evaluated every single second, but it was about the Marines as a whole and about the men you would be laying down your lives for.

There was one man in our platoon who was always dragging us down, while we worked night and day to turn ourselves into elite Marines. Unsurprisingly, he was on everyone's shit list. One morning in the middle of summer, as we were getting dressed at our bunks in preparation for another normal day on the range, he fell down the wall and grabbed and activated the fire alarm while he was trying to stabilize himself.

The sergeants ordered everyone to get out of the barracks, so the fire department could show up and make sure everything was in order, and that there was no risk to the rest of the camp. The first responders quickly realized there was no blaze or smoke, and told our superiors one of the recruits had accidentally set off the alarm. The sergeants were furious; now they were out for blood, so they sent us to the sandpit. This wasn't one of the sandboxes I had played in with my sister as a kid; these were for "incentive training," or I.T.—a nice phrase for endless rounds of push-ups, jumping jacks, runs, or any other form of physical torture the sergeants could dream up. To make things worse, it was the middle of summer in South Carolina, and most days it was a relentless 90 degrees with 90 percent humidity, which you couldn't escape, even when you were in the barracks. The sergeants made us run out to the pit and forced us to do every kind of exercise they could throw our way, while the sweat pooled in our underwear and bugs flew around us, biting every exposed part of our bodies they could find. We were pissed at the clumsy idiot who had destroyed our time at the range just because he couldn't look after himself, and turned our day into one filled with pain.

It seemed like we were in the pit forever. I couldn't remember how long we had our noses in the sand with the instructors screaming at us and the fluids rapidly draining from our bodies out of every sweat gland. Just before I passed out from exhaustion, one of the leaders told us to stop and drag ourselves back to the barracks. At the barracks, one of the drill instructors lined us up, looking like he wanted to punish us even further until we wouldn't be able to walk. He still didn't know who had pulled the fire alarm, and he wanted to know so he could single that boot out.

Then, he said: "You know what. We're not going to even deal with this stuff. You deal with it yourselves." Then he walked out and left us all looking at each other, wondering what to do next. All of us were exhausted, but we still had enough energy to take our fury out on whoever was responsible for our suffering. The squad leader and I caught each other's eyes and nodded. The recruit who was consistently letting us down needed to be taught a lesson, one way or another, so I punched him in the face. He was a big bastard, but I dropped him like a sack of bricks. It was wrong, but something had to be done to let this guy know what he'd done was wrong. Two days later they made me squad leader, because they must have liked what I was doing, and soon after, the recruit—who will remain nameless—dropped out for getting a poor evaluation and failing on the range. Parris Island doesn't take any prisoners. After boot camp, we went to infantry school and started to learn more about what was needed to be a Marine. We were starting to think about deployments and where in the world we might end up. It was 2000, and we had no idea where we would end up, but we also had no idea that in eighteen months our world would be completely turned upside down.

In December I was sent to the Twentynine Palms Marine Base in the California desert for my second trip to the west coast, after the church mission when I was seventeen. The name was hilarious, because it was in the middle of the Mojave Desert: there were no trees and nothing grew there. The base covered more than 931 miles—three times the size of New York City—and had around 20,000 Marines living there. It was the biggest training facility in the U.S. where you can train ground and air units at the same time, and had a mock Afghan village with a mosque, people dressed as locals, and an "IED Valley" where infantrymen can learn how to spot and defend themselves from attacks. The desert heat was unforgiving, and the filthy water-sewage treatment center nearby, which collected the waste from all the Marine bathrooms, made the whole place stink of shit.

While we were there, my platoon commander sat me down and said that every infantryman needed a specialty when they deployed. He laid down all the options: "Do you want to be an assault climber? Do you want to be a motorman and work with engines? Do you want to be a scout swimmer?" I had been hitting the gym hard and was in great shape, so I didn't want to be stuck in an engineering role, and the assault climbers spend their days on mountains in West Virginia, but I really wanted to travel farther and see more of the country. Even as a kid I hated water. I would dip my toes in at the beach or paddle in the lakes in Ohio, but would have never considered trawling through the freezing water for mile after mile. But then I found out the scout swimmer school was in Cocoa Beach, Florida, and even though I hated water I thought to myself, *The beaches and the sun sound pretty awesome.* The commander even told me it wasn't as much of a workout, but he played me for the fool I was. Five days a week we ran three miles with a pack to the pool, then swam for two miles, and then ran back. I was so drained each day that when we finished, I would eat everything I could to refuel, and then sleep for eighteen hours until the next morning, when we would have to do it all over again. It was jog, swim, run, eat, rest, repeat for five months—and by the end of it, I could run sixteen miles without even thinking about it or falling out of line.

Alongside the endless laps of the pool or miles in the sea, we did recon missions to replicate assaulting a beach. The swimmers would approach the sand, and the trailing Marine battalion could come in on their boats to attack. One day, when I was 550 yards out to sea, I took out a knife when I saw what I thought was a shark swimming thirty yards away from me, like in a scene from *Jaws*. I noticed the fin do a ninety-degree turn straight toward me, then sink as though it was ready to pounce and turn me to mincemeat. I had never been so scared in my life. I thought I was going to die, and I was ready to defend myself. The beast was about ten feet away from me when I realized it was a dolphin. I got back to the beach with the rest of the unit, and laughed my ass off while the adrenaline slowly dropped away.

Everyone around us—including the passengers on cruise ships coming in to dock—thought we were Navy SEALS, because we were jetting around in little rubber Zodiac boats with our wetsuits and fake rifles, and by the end of the training we were swimming one kilometer offshore with radios and weapons strapped to us. One of our final missions was an urban beach landing at night without any engines. Being invisible was the key part of the job as a scout swimmer, so the only thing that could be above water was our eyes. All the guys in the unit were connected with hooks attached to a rope known as a Budweiser line. It was pitch black as we approached the landing, and we were invisible. We were swimming with our rubber rifles below the surface of the water, when we noticed a man in a boat in front of us fishing alone. He wasn't involved in the training mission. In a real-world situation, we would have had to check him out and decide whether to open fire or get him to safety. He turned around to reach into his tackle box when he saw the eyes poking out of the water and he froze, so the lieutenant and I got up out of the water and asked him: "Dude, what the fuck are you doing?" He was terrified and almost fell in the water when he reached for the engine to drive away. Our position and the training mission had been compromised by the shouting, so we headed to the beach to debrief and wait for a van to show up to take us back to base. That's when we heard sirens from cop cars roaring towards us and screeching to a halt in the parking lot. The officers got out of their vehicles, guns drawn, and told us to put our hands up and our guns down. The fisherman had called the cops because he thought the guns were real.

"Whoa, whoa," the lieutenant shouted back, and told the officers the guns were rubber and we were from the Department of Defense. Still with their weapons out, they came towards us to make sure we weren't trying to throw them off, like we were a gang of armed robbers. When they realized we were Marines and it was safe, they laughed with us, but we never saw the poor fisherman again after we put the fear of God into him.

I returned to Camp Lejeune in North Carolina after completing basic training, just months before what would be my first deployment in September 2001, and was having the time of my life. I'd had my first beer bong from the second floor of the barracks, having spent most of high school barely touching alcohol. I was in the weight room every hour I had to spare, bulking up to be in the best physical shape of my life, and I was doing what I now felt that God had put me on this earth to do. I was ready to go wherever they wanted to send me, and perform any task thrown my way—but there was still time for a hiccup.

One day after we finished on the range, we decided to spend our downtime messing around in the ocean, before turning in for the night. The Marines were training us to be the most fearsome fighters in the world, but when we had the chance, we acted like children. We would let loose and do everything our parents would be disappointed in. Splashing around as the sun set in North Carolina, we tossed each other in the ocean like rag dolls: we'd place our hands just below the surface to form a platform, get another grunt to stand on our palms, and then we would lift our hands up and throw the grunt into the air so that he slammed back down into the ocean, like we would do in the pool as kids with our dads. We were all laughing and cracking jokes and we didn't care about anything.

One of the Marines with us was a beast. He was six feet, four inches, 250 pounds, and about 3 percent body fat. When it was my turn to be launched, I waded over to him and watched as he lowered his hands and told me to get on. I didn't give it a second thought and pulled my leg up, put my foot down, and put my hands on his shoulders. He shouted, "Three, two, one," and hurled me into the night sky. I flew into the air, still laughing with everyone around me. The water where we were swimming went up to their shoulders, but I was smaller so I could only just keep my head above the water. What I didn't know was that I had been thrown into a spot where it was shallow, and the water only went up to shin height. I was about to fall victim to the first bit of bad luck of my career. It would be the first of many. Sometimes I was very lucky, but this time, as a young Marine less than a year out of graduating high school, it wasn't to be.

I felt the splash of the water on my face, and then a huge impact on my head that I thought was a rock. I blacked out, and it was the first of far too many times when I thought I was dead. I feared I had brought it all to an end just a few months after starting boot camp, going through hell, and finally being on the road to becoming a full-blooded Marine, ready to fight for my country anywhere in the world.

I couldn't move. I was dead weight in the freezing water around me. The guys started screaming, swam towards me, and turned me over so I wouldn't drown. They checked to see if I was conscious and started frantically dragging me out of the water. They didn't know whether I had broken my neck, or my back, or had just suffered a fatal head injury. The guys reacted as if I had been shot in the battlefield, and they wanted to get me to safety while under enemy fire.

They called in a casevac (short for "casualty evacuation"—a team to get me to the nearest medical facility as quickly as possible), and I woke up in hospital in more pain than I had ever experienced in my life, without knowing much about what had happened or how much time I had been unconscious. I was bedridden and groggy and my head was covered in bandages, but all I wanted to do was return to training. My commander also wanted me back out there and stood at the end of my bed, making sure I wasn't overreacting and trying to skip out on the rest of my squad. The officers didn't care about feelings or pain. They were only interested in whether a Marine could stand on two feet, hold a rifle, and pull the trigger in anger.

The nurse got my commander's hint and figured out a way to try and speed up my recovery. She leaned over me and said, "Hey. I'm going to give you something for the pain." She gave me a couple more pills, and then a couple more. Then I woke up in more pain, with still little memory of what had happened. To go with my throbbing head, my cheek was now hurting, and I had no idea why.

"You stopped breathing because of the medication I gave you. So your commander slapped you in the face to get you to wake up." I was terrified that they were just loading me up with painkillers, so I would be out of the hospital and back on the range by the next morning as if nothing had happened. I didn't want to be strapped down and surrounded by medical staff, and miss out on months of 4 a.m. wake-up calls, cleaning the bathroom floors with toothbrushes, runs in the middle of the night, swims in sub-zero waters, ten-mile hikes in the blistering Carolina heat, and getting my orders to serve anywhere in the world on what would have been my first trip out of the United States. Sure enough, the pain subsided, and I went back to the barracks with prescriptions for Percocet and Dilaudid, two very powerful opioids that—years later—would be at the heart of the epidemic sweeping the U.S. Percocet combines oxycodone and acetaminophen, is derived from the same source of morphine as heroin, and targets the brain's reward center to help you deal with pain. I felt great when I took it, and I would find later that—as with most other pain killers—the euphoria is what gets you hooked. Dilaudid isn't much different, yet it was still at my disposal.

I still hadn't been diagnosed with a particular injury, but I was restricted in the training I could do, because they were worried about long-term damage to my neck. To the medical team, my head wasn't the issue. I was barred from the range and most exercises to help me recover, so I went to the gym and concentrated on working out until I was cleared to go back to fighting, which I hoped would be in days, not weeks. The weekend after I was released from the infirmary, I went to get a haircut from the camp barber while jacked up on the pain meds the doctors had given me. I would walk around in a daze and would stumble around the dorms drooling—but I couldn't feel anything. I was high. It was something I had never experienced in my life. It was surreal, but I didn't even think about the incident in the sea, or the long-term damage I may have been doing to myself while swallowing my pills. I had no idea what was going on, and the guys on my team were getting more worried each hour they saw me. When the barber shaved my head, I turned to my roommate and saw he was staring at me wide-eyed, mouth agape.

"Holy shit, dude, what is wrong with your head?" he said.

I looked in the mirror and saw a huge swollen lump on my skull that looked like a football trying to break through the surface of the skin. Confused, and not really processing what was going on, I pressed the bulge down and started laughing.

"I can press down my brain," I said with a slur. I could push the lump so far inward that it would reach the second knuckle on my index finger. I brushed it off and said it just "looked off," so I just went about the rest of my weekend like nothing was wrong, and got ready to get back to work on Monday.

When I showed up to training after a drug-induced sleep, I was sent straight back to the hospital after I showed more people around me, including the instructors, the new party trick I could perform with my head. The doctors ran a series of tests on my head and told me I had a subdural hematoma, and my brain was leaking fluids. The first traumatic brain injury of my career was confirmed, and I hadn't even stepped onto a battlefield. I was pulled from all training, including gym time, and was kept on my painkiller regimen. I had to deal with it; I had come too far to let the injury get in the way, so I kept taking the medication and just waited until my first trip overseas that was scheduled for September, 2001.

CHAPTER 5

It was early September 2001, and I was set to leave on the 18th for a joint training operation with the Egyptians known as Exercise Bright Star, which has happened every two years since 1980 (after the signing of the Camp David Accords in 1978). In the last few months of my training, I had carried on as a scout swimmer in Puerto Rico and the Bahamas. We'd swim to the beach and guard boats, while the Marines came in behind us and completed their mission. The water was so clear you could see the fish swimming on the ocean floor, even when it was fifteen feet deep. A hammerhead got so close to us during one operation, our sergeant reached down and grabbed it straight out of the water, just so he could see what happened.

At that point, I was sure I wouldn't be going to a conflict zone. I was expecting to sail across the other side of the world, to jump around ports, and visit places like Italy and Spain. I had just taken leave to go back to see my family in Ohio. While they were still as dysfunctional as I remembered,

I enjoyed the sense of normalcy, and talking with my sister Kristan about how pumped I was to finally be going on my first trip outside the United States.

I returned to Lejeune on September 10, where the mood was oddly relaxed, considering we were about to be deployed. As the 26th Expeditionary Unit, we were one of the three most prepared units to deploy with the Marine Corps at the time. Our ship was loaded with vehicles, and we were just waiting for leave to finish, so we could hop on and go wherever we were needed. We thought we would be ready for anything.

The morning of September 11, I woke up at 5:00 a.m., and I could already feel the North Carolina heat and humidity through the windows as I got down from my bunk, slipped into my clothes, and headed for the gym like clockwork. I hit the weights with some of my buddies, cracked jokes, and talked about how we imagined the Mediterranean would be full of women in bikinis and yachts. We had only seen the turquoise waters, white beaches, and port towns full of bars and fancy restaurants in movies with our high school girlfriends—of which I had only had one.

I headed to the shower to wash off the sweat and then walked back to my room, where everything seemed normal. Then my roommate Brooks poked his head in the door to see me getting dressed, and said, "Dude, something's happened." He didn't look scared or concerned—just confused.

I followed him into the next room where the radio was tuned to *The John Boy and Billy Big Show*. They were shock jocks who normally played classic rock, made fun of the news, and had everyone in the barracks in hysterics. But this morning, they struck a serious tone. They were reading a developing story coming out of New York, but they weren't really sure what was going on.

"We are hearing that a plane has flown into the World Trade Center," one of the hosts said. I can't remember which one. Brooks and I looked at each other in shock. It sounded like an accident, and one of us cracked a joke about low-flying aircraft. Everyone thought a small prop plane had flown into the tower. Could the pilot have had a heart attack?

We sat and listened, waiting for more information to clear up the situation. Then we heard there was live feed of the Twin Towers on every TV news channel, so we turned on *The Today Show*, to watch what the rest of America and the world was seeing while eating their breakfasts, getting ready for work, and sending their kids off to school.

Ten seconds later, the second plane flew straight into the South Tower, live on the TV in front of us. That moment will forever be seared into my memory because in seconds, my career in the Marines changed. The plane wasn't small. It had the wingspan of a Boeing passenger jet, and it smashed into the building with such ferocity that I thought I could feel the impact. This was no accident. We were under attack. It was real.

"Holy shit, something's going down. We're getting hit," my buddy said. Our instincts to respond and fight back made us jump up.

Sergeant Muniz came sprinting down from the company office yelling, "2nd Platoon, form up!" We hauled our asses downstairs ready to receive orders. He told us that the Pentagon and the Marine Corp didn't really know what was going on. They didn't know who had hit us or why. Around that time, one of George W. Bush's aides was whispering in his ear, while he was reading to elementary school children in Florida. Muniz said the base was going to be put on lockdown in fifteen minutes. No one would be allowed in or out, because we could be deployed at any moment to respond to whichever bastard had done this to us.

"If you have family in town, this could be one of the last times you will see them," Muniz said. "If you don't, then this could be one of the last chances of freedom before they send us out to wherever we need to go."

He didn't tell us what to do, but we knew he was saying that we had a small window to try to leave before the shit really hit the fan. I assumed the training operation with the Egyptians would be cancelled, and the cruise across the Mediterranean would be replaced with a battlefield face-off against whoever was responsible.

My fellow Marine Pete Schuster had a car, so we hopped in with another friend and sped towards the gates of Lejeune and tried to head off base. The speed limit was twenty miles per hour, and the military police on base will pull over anyone. But they ignored our speeding and let us pass. They knew what was happening, and let us leave as quickly as possible. By that point, the Pentagon had also been hit by another plane. The U.S. had just been victim to the worst attack on its homeland in history, and we were going to be the first ones out there fighting back.

We didn't do anything when we got off base. We just stayed in the house of a Marine who had family nearby, and waited for news. We didn't get drunk, we didn't meet up with girls, we didn't go to a bar. There were no clichés and no thoughts of "This is our last night on Earth, so what shall we do?" We just sat by our phones, standing by for our orders. Our eyes were glued to the TV, watching the endless coverage of smoke plumes filling the skies above Manhattan, with New Yorkers running for their lives covered in dust and debris. Every single one had pure terror on their face. They were in suits and ties and pencil skirts, screaming for their loved ones, as they ran past lines of fire trucks and cop cars with their sirens on, for all the news channel sound crews to hear. I tried to imagine the pure fear and terror they were feeling, while the world was watching through its fingers and through tears in its eyes. What floor were they on when a plane hit their tower? Who were they thinking of? I had never been to New York, but I had always dreamed of what it would be like. What was unfolding in front of me was Armageddon—an event of such magnitude it was impossible to fathom. It was a darkness that I had never seen and didn't think was ever possible.

The attack on 9/11 was when I realized how much hatred is in the world. Watching coverage of first responders picking through the rubble of Ground Zero, trying desperately, and with a sliver of hope, to find anyone alive, and seeing the celebrations going on throughout the Middle East and Asia filled me with a fury beyond words.

I watched President Bush tell America that terrorism against our nation would not stand, and when he vowed to hit back with full force, I silently did the same. It may sound cold and callous, but at that moment, I thought about executing every person celebrating the 9/11 attacks, and I would have done it with a smile on my face. To this day, the images from 9/11 are among the few things on this Earth that can bring a tear to my eye. Marines were late coming home from leave, because they were helping pull people out of the rubble, with hundreds of New York cops and firefighters. They stayed in apartments overlooking Ground Zero for weeks, and spent every day sifting through the snapped steel beams, the molten office furniture, and the disintegrated concrete, for signs of life. For months after 9/11, there were still fires at the crash site and fears that more buildings could collapse. I had friends that lost family in the towers.

We stayed by our phones as more details surfaced about who was responsible. All signs coming from the White House pointed to a small group of terrorists in Afghanistan, who hated America and wanted to wage jihad on the U.S. We still didn't know where we were going, but we were mentally preparing for the mountains of South West Asia and the "Graveyard of Empires."

Our panicked families kept calling us, trying to figure out the next move and the fate that awaited us. Kristan was in a seminary in Louisville, Kentucky, and was trying to get in touch with me. She knew, as soon as she saw the second plane hit, that I was going to end up somewhere she didn't want to imagine. As kids we had faced the world on our own, and she knew that my passion was being in the Marines, but for the first time in our lives, we faced the prospect of being on different sides of the world and in a far different reality than the fields in Rust Belt Ohio.

On September 12, after less than twenty-four hours away, we got the call to come back to Camp Lejeune. Our September 18 deployment would proceed on schedule, and we were still going to travel to the Mediterranean for our operation with the Egyptians, but we all knew that it probably wouldn't be our final destination.

We loaded up on the ship, and headed across the Atlantic for a few days of freedom in Italy and Spain, where we enjoyed a drink and kept waiting for developments.

We were near the end of our training in Egypt, when we were suddenly told the ship would be leaving earlier—on October 7. It would be the same day President Bush told the nation, from the Oval Office, that the U.S. military was going into Afghanistan. Al Qaeda and the Taliban were the targets, and Osama Bin Laden was now the most wanted man in the world. We were going to be one of the first Marine units on the ground. B-52s had been bombing Taliban frontlines in southern Afghanistan for months and had been helping the rebels in the north fight back and gain ground. I was trained to be a scout swimmer. I'd spent most of the last two years in the water storming and securing beaches, and my first deployment would be to a landlocked, mountainous country. We sailed up the Suez Canal, and trained by running sixteen one-mile laps of the ship's flight deck.

As the departure moved closer, we suddenly received orders we were changing to a smaller boat. The Pentagon had passed on intelligence that there was a Chinese merchant vessel nearby, and one of Osama Bin Laden's children was on board. It was what we had been waiting for: we had reached the war. There weren't many details. We only knew that there was a possibility that a kid of the man who orchestrated the attack on America was hiding somewhere on the ship, and we had to prepare. I was excited that I was finally able to channel some of the fury I had been holding in from that day, and do what I felt I was born to do.

Senior officers sat our platoon down, and told us we would be performing a search and seizure with the Navy and the SEALs. Another Marine unit would have usually been tasked to do the raid, but they had been held up near the horn of Africa, so it was up to our team to get it done. I had never been trained to attack a boat, and it was the first time I was given combat orders. It was my first mission, and I wasn't going to fuck it up. I was also told that this was the first time I could end up pulling the trigger in anger at an enemy combatant. It was time to get my affairs in order. At just nineteen years old, I prepared my will and wrote my first death letter.

Having to write down everything you want to say to your family and friends is disquieting. What are you supposed to say? "Sorry, Mom." "I love you, Dad." "I'll always remember our church group trips and hunting snakes in Ohio, Kristan." I can no longer recall what I wrote, but I remember none of the Marines penning these letters had dry eyes by the end of it. It was the first time I imagined what would happen if I never saw my family again, and their final memory of me would be a scribbled handwritten letter, handed over by a Marine knocking at the door. I knew I would have to write that letter at some point in my career, but I never imagined it would be this quickly—just over a year after graduating high school, and three months after I had left the United States for the first time.

I addressed the goodbye letters to my parents, my sister, and my best friends from the high school band, and then signed my will as the countdown to the operation continued. I went through all the outcomes of the mission in my head, and tried to calibrate all of my training for an operation I may never have been involved in, had the circumstances been different. I was about to be one of the first American troops to get a chance to get back at Bin Laden. Capturing one of his children would be a major victory and a dent in morale for the head of Al Qaeda, who had a huge family—at least twenty children by four different wives.

Just a few days earlier, President Bush had confirmed that he had given the military orders to strike Al Qaeda military installations and disrupt communications, after the Taliban refused to meet demands to close down terrorist training camps and return any Americans they had unjustly detained. Bin Laden released a speech on the same day, calling the United States hypocrites, and saying Muslims were using violence to respond to eighty years of humiliation. Our families back home now knew where we were going, but mine didn't know that I was in the middle of the Arabian Sea, in the dead of night, ready to enter the war far earlier than I could have imagined. I was ready, but holy shit, was it real.

We gathered our gear, armed up, and stayed awake through the night, waiting for the call to go. Just after 1 a.m., we were given the all-clear, and the adrenaline started flowing. I looked out over the pitch-black waters from the deck of the ship, and could barely make out the lights on the target vessel. The air was still, and there was an unnerving silence until the Seahawk helicopter rotor blades spun to life. They were so quiet that the enemy wouldn't know that a forty-seven-million-dollar, twin-engine attack helicopter was hovering above them, until it was too late. I was part of the second wave of the attack, so I watched as the first set of helicopters sped off into the night, and headed for the boat on the horizon. As my second wave left, I held on as the pilot launched us off the deck. The Marines around me were quiet as mice and laser-focused on getting the job done. Just two minutes later, the pilot stopped, suspended above the ship that from so high up looked like a matchbox. I hooked myself into a rappel line, leaned backwards out of the door with my back hanging over the landing skids, and got ready to drop. I steadied myself, closed my eyes for a brief second, and then inhaled some of the ocean air around me. Before that moment, I had only ever rappelled at boot camp—when I was twenty feet up, the conditions were controlled, and I knew what awaited me when I landed.

I pushed off the helicopter into the black abyss, and plummeted towards the vessel. The rope slipped through my hands without any resistance. I peered over my left shoulder and watched as the deck got closer to me by the second. I could see Marines breaking through the door of the bridge, but one had stayed back and was on his knee looking like he had been hit. Then it hit me—I was dropping into combat.

I braced for the impact of the landing, and kept looking around to try and figure out what was going on. *Where was this kid hiding? Was he even on board? Were we in a gunfight? How many of them were there? What firepower did they have? Were they trained?* I tried to remember all the training scenarios from Camp Lejeune, Pendleton, and Cocoa Beach so I could adapt without hesitation.

When my feet hit the deck, it was like I had landed on black ice, with the wash from the rotor blades. A corpsman was standing at the bottom to make sure we didn't slip. My feet were sliding everywhere, and he shouted at me "go that way" while pointing at the bridge as I tried to regain my bearings. I ran to the bridge on orders to hold it down with my platoon commander, while other teams searched every inch of the ship.

We stayed there all day, waiting for confirmation that one of the children of the world's most wanted terrorist was stowed away, trying desperately to evade capture, but the operation turned up nothing. I later learned the Marine I saw clutching his knees hadn't been shot. He had felt a flash of heat when one of the Chinese crew members jumped out of a hatch and threw coffee on him, making him believe he had been hit.

All they found on the ship were mountains of rice. There was nothing suspicious, and no members of the Bin Laden family were on board, as far as we knew. While the result was disappointing—given I'd been ready to open fire at any enemy—at least I had my first mission under my belt. The Marines around me also felt more comfortable, now that we knew what was expected of us. It showed that we were going to knock down any door, board any ship, or hit absolutely anywhere, if there was even the slightest chance we could catch someone close to him. It was my first involvement in what would become America's longest war, and we hadn't even reached Afghanistan.

We kept running laps as we waited for our next orders and headed further into the Arabian Sea, when one day we were told to gather on the deck. I had no idea what was going on. We'd had no heads-up about any operation, and I knew we would get advanced notice if we were going to fly into southern Afghanistan where the Taliban had concentrated most of their fighters, and where the airstrikes were focusing their firepower. We learned from our families that the news was wall-to-wall coverage of explosions in the mountains, and bomb craters surrounded by mud huts.

We were called onto the deck, to see a shipment the Pentagon had flown in from Ground Zero. There was part of a girder from one of the towers and a Star-Spangled Banner that had been hanging inside when they came down. What I saw on the deck was proof that my trip to Afghanistan was my destiny. Every reason I had to fight was right in front of me. I was awestruck by how the enormous steel beam had bent and broken under the weight of all the floors that collapsed above it. The flag was burned around the edges and had small tears, but was still mostly intact. I signed the girder with the rest of my platoon, and took photos in front of the flag. We were all grinning like idiots as we posed for the cameras, but the moment was so powerful. It connected us with all the rescuers still searching through the rubble for survivors, working day and night to make sure anyone holding onto life was found. I had spent my life preparing to become a Marine, and I knew that my mission was to avenge the New Yorkers picking up the pieces of their beloved city, and the more than three thousand people killed by Al Qaeda that day. We were about to wreak havoc on Al Qaeda and the Taliban.

CHAPTER 6

It was December 22 when we got the thumbs up that our journey through the Arabian Sea was coming to an end, and we were heading into southern Afghanistan, after taking off from Pasni in Pakistan. Our entrance was like the opening scene from *Apocalypse Now*, one of the war movies I had watched as a kid, when the soldiers are leaning out of helicopters over Vietnamese rice fields. I looked out of the window of our helicopter, and saw a line of thirty aircraft flying level with the top of the jagged mountains in the background. Inside them was immense firepower: millions of dollars of ammunition and rockets, and some of the fiercest and most-highly trained warriors in the world. Beneath them was a vast landscape with snow-covered peaks, deep gorges, winding valleys and small patches of fertile land, where farmers harvested heroin and tended to their animals.

We landed at Camp Rhino, an airstrip in the Registan Desert that had been seized a month earlier—on November

15—by the 15th Marine Expeditionary Unit, who were the first conventional force on the ground to help pave the way for the onslaught to follow. It was the first of many land bases the U.S. set up during Operation Enduring Freedom, and was the starting point for the initial combat operations in Helmand and Kandahar. The base—which had previously been a place for Arab birdwatchers to keep their falcons—was freezing, windy and sparse, with only a handful of buildings and a runway.

As my plane touched down, I noticed craters from U.S. strikes to take over the base were still smoking. A couple days after our arrival, we packed into a tiny hangar for a USO show with performances by Dallas Cowboys cheerleaders, comedian Drew Carey, and singer Neil McCoy. The show offered one final morale boost before we were thrown into chaos, marking the last time we could kick back and enjoy ourselves for months. McCoy rocked it and played us some new songs. Carey had us laughing with jokes he could only get away with in front of a crowd of men, repeatedly saying he knew we would rather see the cheerleaders than his "fat ass."

During the show, we heard a special forces recon team was returning with the first prisoner to be captured during the War on Terror. I was stunned when I heard he was American. It was John Walker Lindh, the "American Taliban." He had been with a unit of non-Afghan soldiers when the American bombing campaign began, and he was forced to retreat and then surrender to the Northern Alliance. There was a fire-fight at the fortress he was moved to—at Qala-i-Jangi on the outskirts of Mazar-i-Sharif—which killed CIA officer Mike Spann and hundreds of prisoners. Lindh spent a few days huddled in a basement, hiding, and when he managed to get above ground, he was handed over to U.S. Special Forces. I heard rumors at Camp Rhino that he had links to Al Qaeda and had met Bin Laden.

One of the guys in our company had a brother in the recon team escorting Lindh, and asked the rest of us: "Hey, do you want to see him?"

"Hell yeah, I want to see him," I said. Really, I just wanted to get my hands on him and beat him to within an inch of his life. When we saw Lindh, he was tied to a chair in a base building, wearing a jumpsuit with a giant "P" across the chest and a bag over his head. We wanted to get closer, to smell him and give him a taste of what we felt he deserved as a traitor to his country. But we kept our hands off and went back to enjoy the rest of the show, like nothing had happened.

We were only at Rhino for three days before being told we were moving out, as the Pentagon brass formulated new ground operations aimed at forcing the Taliban to retreat even further. Our company was going to catch the ninety-minute flight northeast to Kandahar Airport, at the center of the jihadi's "spiritual birthplace." The insurgents took control of the city in 1994, made it their "capital," and imposed strict sharia law on all the residents, including the banning of traditional education for boys and girls, watching TV, and playing sports. The Navy had already been hitting targets occupied by the Taliban from the Persian Gulf, and we were going in to maintain control of the airport and surrounding areas.

As we flew over the mountains, I kept hearing a quiet "pop" from the C-130 engines. A senior officer next to me laughed when I asked what the noise was.

"Dude. Those are rounds," he said. "Those are from the Taliban hidden in the hills. Don't worry, it's the first time I've been shot at too, but those rounds can't do anything. They are just ricocheting off the bottom of the plane. None of the artillery from those Soviet guns can break through. There's no need to be nervous."

I was nervous, but also impressed that fighters—with far less skill and training—could hit a plane thousands of feet up, with an AK-47. Our equipment was far more advanced, but their instincts, and the skills they had picked up in camps around the country, meant they were a threat—a threat I would encounter far too closely on more than one occasion, on my tours in this backward country.

My company was told we would be securing the perimeter at the airfield. They were still setting up the base and members of all the military branches were arriving every day. Just after I landed, I went outside to smoke a cigarette, and saw a huge guy with a long red beard, in camo, who was armed to the teeth. I approached him and asked who he was with.

"I can't tell you that," he said with a smile.

I started laughing and asked again: "No, seriously dude, what unit are you in?" He looked back at me with a more serious expression and didn't answer. He must have had top secret clearance, way above my pay grade. He must have been a member of the special ops teams who were performing operations in the surrounding hills against the Taliban, while the conventional troops on the ground were increasing in numbers.

Our battalion's job was security. We would be stationed just outside the airport fence and keep an eye on any approaching militants, or check to see if civilians were a threat. Our first job was to dig fighting holes. The ground was so hard our shovels would barely get past the surface, so we had to bring in combat engineers to use explosives to blast five-foot craters for our positions.

For months, the holes served as our home for eight mind-numbingly boring hours a day, staring into nothing. I had thought I would be thrown straight into the action as soon as I landed, with raids and nighttime operations but everyone had to do a job, and ours was—in my opinion—the worst. I spoke to the same two people for months, during the shifts that were either in hundred-degree stifling heat during the day or bone-shattering cold at night. The only thing that saved me from complete boredom was a book I stole from the library; we weren't technically allowed to bring them into the holes, but reading only kept me occupied for so long. We just kept looking into the mountains. Sometimes we could see Afghans perched on the hillside, drawing our positions and trying to strategize, but they were so far away they weren't really a threat, and we couldn't do anything because of the rules of engagement. The area around the airport was also littered with landmines left over from the Soviet Union in the 1970s, so we couldn't advance out of the holes without putting ourselves at danger or using metal detectors to make sure the path was safe. There were only small strips of white tape you could follow where engineers had determined the area was clear of explosives. When I was clearing my fighting hole one day, I noticed what looked like a Pepsi can thrown on the ground next to some sheet metal. I pointed it out to Hall—one of our corpsmen—and Staff Sergeant Muniz, by putting my foot on it. Muniz started running over to me with his eyes bulging out of his head, grabbed me by the collar, and shouted: "Bee, you dumbass. That's a fucking mine." It was a Soviet OZM-72 bounding frag mine. I was still standing on the can, didn't move a muscle, and was petrified that—during a tour with virtually no action—I would get killed for being an idiot. We called in EOD (Explosive Ordnance Disposal) and they arrived within fifteen minutes—the quickest response time I had ever heard of. They had balls of steel and a swagger unlike anyone else in the U.S. military, despite the fact that cutting one wrong wire, or applying pressure where they shouldn't, would end up with their remains being scattered for miles to the point where they couldn't be identified. A member of the team jumped from his Humvee, walked over, looked at the metal for thirty seconds, and told me in his calmest voice to move back a couple of meters. "We'll blow it up just to be sure," he said. He pulled what looked like white putty and a green plastic wrap out of his daypack, started laying sandbags around the mine, prepared the charge for the controlled explosion, and told me; "Watch how far I can launch this thing." I retreated even further towards the fence line when the EOD radio operator said, "Controlled det" (controlled detonation), and shouted, "Popping smoke!" I got crouched down in my fighting hole as they started counting down from thirty seconds. There was then a huge *whoomp* sound and a wave of energy coursed through my body, like nothing I had ever experienced. Then I lifted my head and watched as a sandbag on top of the mine flew more than a hundred feet in the air, and landed with a thump a hundred yards away. It wouldn't be the last time being a dumbass could have gotten me killed. It was a trait I would never seem to kick as a grunt—much to the despair of my family, friends, and colleagues, especially those who had to save my ass.

Journalists covering the opening of Operation Enduring Freedom would sometimes lean in and talk to us, with their press flak jackets and helmets, and ask what we were doing. That was the only real entertainment we had. Every so often farmers would cross our sightlines with emaciated cows, or families walking across would stop and peer at us with curiosity. They were people whose country had been torn apart by decades of conflict, corruption, hunger, and poverty, and you could see it in their faces, through binocular lenses.

One of the only times we could leave the line was to shit, and we didn't have the luxury of a porta-potty. Each platoon had its own giant tractor tire, where they would do their business and set it on fire, a couple of times a day. The horrific smell became part of my daily routine.

I thought the whole of my first tour was going to be sitting in a hole and doing nothing while the rest of our forces were taking it to the Taliban. I was frustrated. I wanted action, and to do my part against evil. Then came the night of January 6, 2002.

I was the radio operator on the night shift. It was cold as hell, and as quiet as it had been most other evenings. I just sat and looked up into the sky full of stars, which was one of the only positives of being on duty after sunset. It was around 1:00 a.m. when a plane took off and roared overhead. It was a monster C-141 Starlifter, a plane so big it could carry multiple tanks. I watched as it soared above, when I suddenly heard what sounded like popcorn in a microwave. I started laughing, and turned around to the guys in the battalion and said:

"Who the hell brought a popcorn machine out here?" That was the only thought that crossed my mind until my battalion commander ran and jumped into my hole, snatched the radio from out of my hand, and started screaming into it. He was frantic and telling me to get down, but we still had no idea what was going on.

Then I heard him tell the operator he had seen someone in the hills firing an RPG at the plane while it was taking off, but it had misfired and the sparks had caused the crackling sound. The commander turned around, found a spot on the mountain, and opened fire with full fury. I began to shake so hard from adrenaline that I couldn't control my hands, as I desperately tried to put on my night vision goggles. There were four or five fighters firing directly at us, and the only thing I could see were the muzzle flashes on the hillside. I finally got the damn goggles on, grabbed my gun, and unloaded my magazine straight with the rest of the platoon peppering the mountain. The militants on the hill probably weren't expecting that kind of response. There were thirty of us in those holes, and for many of us, it was our first firefight. The ground around us was covered in empty casings, and you could smell the firepower over the stench of the shit coming from the tire. We each unloaded a magazine, the opposite of what you should be doing in that situation, but the excitement got to us. We were a bunch of Marines barely out of high school, finally able to fire their weapons, fueled by the anger that had been building in the weeks since the attacks, weeks spent waiting patiently on boats, or in our bunks on bases, for the call telling us we would be heading to Afghanistan.

The fighters ran into a mud hut to hide from the hail of rounds. The huts were the size of garden sheds but had thick walls that could protect them from the gunfire. So the senior officers brought in a LAV-25 Light Armored Vehicle from our unit, with a twenty-millimeter Bushmaster cannon that fired rounds the size of Red Bull cans, perched on the top. It slowly rolled up beside our holes, and I watched as they maneuvered the barrel into position. I knew what would happen next.

They opened fire with the cannon and destroyed the mud hut, and everyone inside it. The platoon started screaming and yelling with excitement as it kept firing. After a few minutes, the return fire had stopped, and that was the end of my first real face-off with enemy combatants. It was over in what felt like seconds, but it was what I had been preparing for. I had experienced the rush of live fire, and the fear that fills up inside you when you are forced to rapidly respond. No training can prepare you for that. Nothing in life even matches. Then the energy died down, we settled back into our holes, and watched the sun rise on another day of sitting around doing nothing.

Later, we learned the plane was full of a hundred shackled prisoners, heading to a new camp at Guantanamo Bay, where terror suspects and militant enemy combatants were being detained under the harshest conditions. The camp had only been open for a short time and no one knew the full extent of what the U.S. was doing inside, but the hunt for Al Qaeda—and any known affiliates in Central Asia—was intensifying, so the detainee count was increasing by the day. We also found out there had been forty insurgents in the hills firing at us, and they had disappeared after the rockets hit their huts. Marines sent out in the aftermath to search for them couldn't find anything or anyone, but the risk was still there.

After the firefight and during the search around the base, Associated Press reporter Ellen Knickmeyer leaned into my hole—during another non-eventful watch shift—to ask me what had happened. As a nineteen-year-old grunt from the Rust Belt, I didn't think the press would be interested in talking to me, but America and the world were keeping close eyes on all the developments on the ground, and every day there were dozens of stories being printed about the opening stages of the Afghanistan War. Little did we know that twenty years later, the U.S. would still be there.

The firefight on that night in January was the only action I would see for the next four months. I would sleep, eat, sit in the hole on the front lines for a few hours, sometimes see an Afghan family or a farmer walking in the distance, leave and sleep again, for days on end. Sometimes our battalion would hike in the mountains, and every so often we would patrol the perimeter fence, but I didn't fire another shot. We hadn't even seen the faces of the Taliban men we were trying to gun down that night. I was bored and I wanted action, but there was nothing, nothing at all. I got a combat ribbon for that night, but there wasn't anything else to show for my first deployment other than a few jokes with the rest of my squad, and stories we were hearing of what was going on in the rest of the country. The start of the invasion crippled Al Qaeda and forced it to retreat, and the Army—with the help of the local militia—began to topple the Taliban regime, so we could start setting up our own democratic government. President Bush had promised to hit the 9/11 perpetrators hard, and he did—I just hadn't been involved. In March 2002 came the start of Operation Enduring Freedom and the blitz to try and completely eradicate the Taliban, in a mission that western forces thought would only take a few months. By then I had been taken off the frontlines to a tented area at Kandahar, to decompress for a few weeks. I spent the rest of my first deployment working out, in an attempt to rebuild the muscle mass I'd lost over months sitting in those holes.

The only showers we'd had in weeks were with baby wipes, so we were desperate to feel hot water again. We asked the Army's 101st Airborne Division if we could use theirs, but they said no. The rivalry between the Army and the Marines was still in full swing, even though we were fighting the same enemy. We were pissed, and just desperate to wash, so we figured out ways to get back at them, when their flag went missing. It was a huge deal. Every division had their own colors and brought them wherever they went, so they could display them on a pole in the middle of the base. The Army launched a health and comfort inspection as an excuse to try and track it down. The check is supposed to evaluate your personal belongings, to check if you are living hygienically—which we weren't at the time—but officers went through every bag, every pack, and every tent, trying to find the flag. They spent hours turning over the barracks and it never showed up. I never knew what really happened to it, but rumors on the base spread that a Marine had buried it somewhere in the desert. Whoever knew the truth was never going to say anything, and was probably saving it as a story to one day tell their grandkids: about how they screwed over the Army because it wouldn't share.

By April 2002 I was on my way home. We had been scheduled to get involved in Operation Anaconda—the name for the first part of the invasion—but whatever mission we were supposed to be sent on was handed over to the Army's 82nd Airborne Division. Our time was up, and we were finally getting out of the desert. Our unit flew out, got on the first available ship, and started weaving our way back to the United States, through the Middle East and Europe. We stopped in Bahrain, and then headed to Aviano Air Base, fifty miles north of Venice. We traveled down to the city and experienced something I never thought I would, after years of taking vacation in Pennsylvania.

We paid a tour guide—funded by the USO—twenty dollars to show us around. We only had to check in with them twice a day, so we got to do our own thing. I saw glassblowing and got to stay in a swanky hotel that would have otherwise cost hundreds of dollars a night. I was only there for forty-eight hours, but I knew straight away that if I ever started a family, I would be bringing them back to experience the magic. I bought a painting of the Bridge of Sighs, which still hangs on my wall. I was taken aback by the architecture and the detail in the white limestone, and watched while the gondolas floated beneath. It would have been so peaceful had it not been for the tourists, but its magic inspired me.

We stopped off again in Rota, Spain, before heading back across the Atlantic to see our families for the first time since 9/11. I had only gotten to speak to my parents and my sister a few times. Our family hadn't changed, but America had. There was a new wave of patriotism, and pure fury and resentment towards anyone who wanted to hurt the United States. More than three thousand people had died in the Twin Towers, but there were millions of victims, and the Marines and the rest of the armed forces were avenging them. We were the heroes acting on behalf of a nation in mourning.

The boat docked in Morehead City, North Carolina, around an hour away from Camp Lejeune. We were close to home, and I was excited knowing that it wouldn't be long between stepping on American soil and getting the chance to hug my family once again. The Marines hired a couple of buses to drive us back along North Carolina Route 24. As we drove out of the base and onto the highway, I looked out of the window, just waiting for the trip to be over, when I noticed there were no other vehicles on the road. A cop car drove in front of us to escort us back, and the road was lined with people. They were cheering for us and waving American flags. Mothers had babies in their arms, and veterans in uniforms saluted, as we made the trip back. For almost an hour, there were barely any stretches of road where there wasn't a crowd waving and smiling back at us. It was a solid line of people welcoming us back, thanking us for what we had done, and it was cool as hell. They had no idea I had only been in one firefight, but they were thankful for the fact that we were out there protecting them. The thought of another attack was still in the air, and at that time the War on Terror was seen as a way of stopping it.

My dad, Grandma Bee, my aunt Jude, and my uncle Steve came to meet me off the bus, and took me to a restaurant to get a proper meal inside me. I talked about sitting in the fighting hole for hours on end, the night we shot at the Taliban, and my adventures through Europe. I had months of memories and almost all good. I walked up to the bar to grab another drink—one of many that afternoon—and my uncle Steve came up to me. He had served in Vietnam, and for thirty years had never spoken about what had happened. It was a trait of a lot of veterans who'd taken on the Vietcong, to not talk about the experiences, but he put his arm around me and shared what he had gone through. I can't remember the details of what he said, but I knew his opening up to me was something out of the ordinary, and when I went back to the table, my stunned father told me, "I've known that man for decades and he has never done anything like that. Until you deployed, he never said a word to anyone about Vietnam."

I spent two weeks in Ohio on post-deployment leave, catching up with my four friends from school, and went to visit my sister at her seminary school in Kentucky, where she was living with her husband. We even got to spend the day at the Kentucky Derby. Both my mom's side of the family and my dad's side of the family had welcome home parties, but most of the time I was just ready and waiting to get back out there. Soon enough, I was back in North Carolina, getting ready for my next orders. We were shifted from a battalion landing team to the 4th Marine Expeditionary Brigade, a new unit that was set up on October 29, 2001, to serve as an anti-terrorism battalion. It was all part of how the Marines were adapting to the War on Terror. We would be ready to be sent out anywhere in the world, with all the assets we needed to deal with terrorist combatants.

The deployment rotation was three months out at an embassy and then six months back. It caused a lot of marriages to break up. We found out we would be stationed at the U.S. Embassy in Kabul. They needed a larger unit of more battle-ready Marines to stand guard and be ready to respond to any threats. The capital city at the time was away from the fight between western forces and the Taliban in the south, but was still a target. Any damage to the embassy would be a significant scalp for the insurgency, so security had to be tight.

It was October 2002, and instead of getting a ship they flew our unit over on commercial flights and through public airports. We walked through the terminals and waited in line to go through security, and board flights with our daypacks and M4 rifles. It was disconcerting, because civilians just awkwardly sat and stared at us. We went to Shannon, Ireland, then on to Bahrain where we spent a couple of weeks, and then finally jetted into Bagram Air Base, forty-three miles outside of Kabul. It was still small, as it had only been a year since British forces had taken it over after a clash between the Taliban and the Northern Alliance, and there were around seven thousand troops from all parts of the world. There was a Pizza Hut, a Subway, an Afghan restaurant, and a Green Beans coffee, but it would be a few years before the Pentagon invested millions turning it into a modern fortress. Taliban prisoners were kept in cages, in an abandoned Soviet warehouse off to the side of the base.

A detachment of Marines from Kilo Battery 3rd Battalion, 11th Marines, and four Marine scout snipers from the 3rd Battalion, 6th Marines, retook the embassy in Kabul in December 2001, after the collapse of the Taliban. They hid in a factory just outside the gates, and arrived on Afghan buses to assault and recapture the outpost that was shut down in 1989. It was still relatively new when we arrived, and the camp was full of high-level State Department officials, including the U.S. Ambassador at the time—Ryan Crocker, CIA officers, and members of Non-Governmental Organizations. The rules of engagement were different from when we were in Kandahar. There, we were told in no uncertain terms not to open fire unless someone was shooting at you. In the embassy, we had the ability to use our firepower more freely, and anything close to the fence was deemed a risk. The Taliban could disguise a bomb as a soccer ball being kicked over the fence. Someone in a window of the houses around you could be a sniper.

But on the weekends, we were allowed to take out the embassy vehicles, and visit the bazaar near the International Security Assistance Force compound. The embassy staff wanted me to train up to start driving the Ambassador around, so they cut me loose with a gunnery sergeant to drive into the middle of Kabul. It was crazy because I had never seen, let alone tried to navigate in, a place like that. There were locals everywhere mingling with representatives and troops from countries around the world. Any of them could have been a member of the Taliban wanting to pick us off or hiding a suicide vest under their robes. I was scared, but I walked around with a little bit of swagger, because I had one deployment under my belt and a feeling of "been there, done that."

We would stroll around the bazaar, with our rifles across our puffed out chests, looking at the tables and stalls full of anything you could want, and it was cheap because they hadn't started inflating prices for the Westerners. I bought a mockup Glock pistol—from 1817, with an ivory handle—for thirty dollars, and my buddies picked up enormous carpets you could ship back home without going through customs checks. It was the chance to send gifts back to our families and keep things for ourselves, from an exotic place for budget prices.

On one of our trips, one of the Marines alongside me—a superhuman looking dude—didn't want to carry his machine gun, so he took out a twelve-gauge shotgun instead. A man came up to the superhuman and started tugging at his sleeve, saying, "Sir, look at this, come look at this. Come, sir." The Afghans can be very touchy-feely people and will try their best to sell you anything. The Marine pushed him off and said, "Dude don't touch me," and we tried to find another route to walk, because we had another two hours before we were due to go back to the embassy. But the man kept following and kept trying to grab his sleeve. The superhuman turned, grabbed hold of him, stared into his eyes, and said again,

"Seriously, stop touching me." The guy—who didn't seem the slightest bit scared—just kept following us, trying to get us to buy whatever shit he was pushing. The superhuman was furious, so he turned around one final time, kicked him in the chest to the ground, and held the twelve-gauge up to his body. The Afghan's eyes turned wide and he put his hands above his head, looking scared to death. He suddenly went quiet, and so did the rest of the bazaar. All the locals around us suddenly dropped to their knees and put their hands over their heads, while staying low to the ground. They were terrified.

"Shit, what do we do?" I said, looking around at the sea of Afghans cowering on the floor. We were there to help them make a living, but the situation in their country was so volatile, they never knew when fighting could erupt. Our rapport with the citizens was growing, but they still saw us as strange visitors. Our squad leader—Sean Morris—told us to wrap up and get back in the van for the compound, like nothing had happened.

My second tour, much like the first, wasn't full of action and we had very limited exposure to the Taliban. An IED blew up inside a trash can just outside the walls, but it wasn't strong enough to do any damage, and a sniper would sometimes hit one of the embassy buildings, but it wouldn't do any damage. Security was tight, and the neighborhood around us was just a bombed-out shell. It looked like a scene from *The Flintstones*: mud huts with holes in them from the endless attacks on the compound over the years. Night-time patrols were spooky. It was pitch-black, and every time we stepped outside, the streets would clear out as if we were cowboys in an old Western, coming into a town with our Stetsons on and our guns drawn. It was nerve-wracking, and you knew you were being watched all the time, whether it was a family peering from their home, or a sniper wanting to do some damage to an exposed unit walking through the streets. But I got out unscathed. We were hit by mortars, but the giant bullet-proof bunkers meant they essentially bounced off. There were too many high-ranking diplomats inside to take any risks.

It was my interaction with the people—who'd had their lives torn apart from decades of Soviet occupation, civil war, and the horrors of the Taliban regime—that would stay with me the most. During one of the weekend trips, we happened to come across an orphanage. We weren't planning on visiting, but just stepped inside to kill some time before we had to go back. There were hundreds of boys and girls inside, lying on beds or on the floor playing with toys. Almost all of them were injured in some way. They had arms or legs missing, or bandages across their faces. Some of them had smiles, the younger ones were crying, but others were just vacantly staring off into the distance. What were they thinking about? Were they reminiscing about the family members they lost? What had happened to them, to make them so deformed? I could feel myself welling up, and worried that we—the U.S.—were responsible for their pain.

I pulled my squad leader to the side while we were walking through one of the wards, and said: "Is this us? Did we do this?"

He calmed me down a little, and told me that the Russians had dropped mines shaped like toys during the 1980s, and some of them were still lying around, or in the ground. During their crackdown before our invasion, the Taliban had also chopped off the limbs of women and girls. It made me more furious. During that horrible thirty-minute trip to the orphanage in Kabul, I had the desire to kill every single member of the Taliban and the Russians who'd put in the mines. How could they do that to innocent little girls, who had done nothing but simply exist? It was an anger I would bring back. I hated them for what they had done to their people, and we were here to stop them and root out the evil.

I was only at the embassy for four months, and there was one enduring experience that I will never forget: the smell of curry. A group of Indian contractors were staying in the compound with us, and every time we went for food in the tiny dining room with the smallest windows, there were two meal choices in the buffet: the day's special, or curry. It was curry for breakfast, lunch, and dinner, and the smell never went away. I still can't stand the smell of curry.

We flew back out again, and headed home without stopping in Europe. My second deployment was under my belt, and I still had only one firefight to my name. I was lucky—I could go back to my family and do the same thing all over again: different welcome home parties with my mom's and my dad's sides of the family, time jerking around with my four friends, and time with my sister. My head was clear, and I still wanted to go back and finish what I considered to be unfinished with the Taliban. What they had done to their people sickened me, and they had moved their country back in time, to something a Western democracy wouldn't even be able to fathom. It would take six years for me to get another shot at the bastards, but as I flew home, I knew I would be back no matter what it took.

CHAPTER 7

On my twenty-first birthday, we started our descent into Guantanamo Bay for my third deployment. The Camp X-Ray detention center was in headlines around the world, and the photos of detainees on their knees in orange jumpsuits—with goggles, earmuffs, and masks, and their hands tied—were what the world associated with it. Because of those images, we called it the Carrot Farm. When we arrived, they were closing down the first prison and setting up a new high-security facility. I didn't know what to expect, as we weren't going to be fighting anyone. The enemy combatants were in the same camp, but were locked up around the clock and were disarmed. There hadn't been any firefights with the Cubans in decades. The barracks on Marine Hill, on the windward side of the island, were pimped out. They had pool tables, and there were two Marines in a room, so it was far more spacious than sleeping in a hangar, and more luxurious than lying in a hole in the desert. My office was right next to the gazebo where Tom Cruise and Jack Nicholson filmed a scene from *A Few Good Men*.

My job was mainly Company Level Intelligence, where we would monitor activity in Cuban airspace, or from one of the posts outside the base, where the Castro regime soldiers were keeping an eye on us. We would send messages to whoever was patrolling the fence line if we received any information. We were the eyes and ears of a base that has always been in a vulnerable position: if the Cubans decided they weren't going to play nice, it could have gotten ugly very quickly, but they never did, and we never had to deal with anything going on outside. I had the dream rotation of one week on post, one week training, and then a week off. For a Marine, it was the life you wanted. We were on a Caribbean island with two of our own bars, and could spend our rest sunbathing or swimming. I could grab a six-pack of beer from the store and sit on the bay, and fish until the sun went down.

I spent most of my time driving up and down the fence line, giving my Marines a break to go to the bathroom and make sure they were fed, and I would inspect their posts to make sure they weren't carrying magazines or books. The Cubans had high-tech cameras that could watch our guys, and if one of them was asleep while on duty, they would send a picture to our intelligence office. So, all they could do was stare at the trees and the sea, if they were lucky enough to get stationed with a view.

The most violence we saw were brawls between Americans. One night at the tiki bar—which looked out over the ocean and was as close as you could get to something straight out of a resort brochure—a few of my platoon were sitting lined up opposite members of the Army. A Marine beside me called Smith, who wasn't tall enough to reach my chin but was hard as nails, suddenly shouted at one of the men: "What did you say to me?" He was older, so we knew that he had a high rank, and I immediately thought to myself: *This is not a good idea.*

There has always been a rivalry between the branches of the military, which seems weird to outsiders, because we are supposed to be fighting together. When tensions flare, it can get nasty, as you want to keep your bragging rights. They were screaming at each other, and stood up like they were inciting us to come and attack.

Smith then picked up a bottle, and—with a one-in-a-million shot—threw it across the bar, and hit the Army guy square in the face. The Army guy started bleeding. Then fists started flying, and everyone at the bar—including the Navy and the Air Force—got involved. Picnic tables were thrown in the air and a couple were set on fire, and there were men rolling around everywhere. It was out of control, and took five minutes until everyone calmed down and ran out of energy. While we were sitting outside the bar, a senior officer came over and told us he could write us up for potential disciplinary action, or we could fix the picnic tables. We spent the week we were supposed to have off sewing pieces of lumber together with twine.

After a few months of what would be my favorite deployment of my time with the Marines, I was on a plane for the shorter flight back to North Carolina for some time at home, and the same routine of welcome home parties and just hanging out, until I got my next orders. I had no motivation to leave the suck, even though some of my buddies were considering getting out—there was still a war to fight, and I still hadn't fulfilled the dreams I had as a child. Recruits and veterans had given the Marines the nickname of "the suck," since American prisoners of war started using it in Vietnam. "Welcome to the suck" is what you hear when you are initiated, and "embrace the suck" is what you hear when you are thinking about giving up. The slang may seem negative, but it is a testament to the dedication and grit of grunts. The idea is to lean into the pain and try to be comfortable, when you are in one of the most uncomfortable situations in your life. I hadn't experienced true pain or discomfort yet, but others had and wanted a way out. But I wanted to be in it for the long haul, and serve my country until I couldn't do it anymore.

When I got back to Lejeune, I was scheduled to return to embassy duty in either Kabul or Djibouti, but for a couple of months I was ordered to stay in the U.S. to do a workup and train Marines who were heading to Afghanistan. At Fort A.P. Hill in Virginia, we used the MILES 2000 laser systems to play what were essentially giant games of laser tag, using blank rounds. The sensors were attached to our gear, equipment, and trucks. If you got hit, you were taken out, or the engine would shut off and the passengers would start beeping. We would take in a team of new arrivals, and go to war with them for hours on end in a mock battle, while I was leading the so-called "enemy." We would attack them from an hour before sunrise, through the whole day and night until the sun came back up. All of the new team were awake the entire time, behind their rifles watching us to see if we would attack. I would have my guys on rotation, so they could pop off a couple of rounds at the arrivals, and then sleep for a few hours. The other team went without sleep for four days, while my Marines were having the time of their lives.

When the training finished, I realized a few years at home may be the best for me, even though I knew I still wanted to see some action. The rotation of the first three deployments had kept me away for too long and it was time to recuperate while I was still serving, so I reenlisted as a recruiter. There was no chance of being deployed, and I could pass on what I had learned to teenagers like me, who had grown up with nothing and needed some direction in their lives. They could travel around the world, get to see European ports, hang out with men their age, and get the chance to kill America's enemies. They would be sent to the most horrendous places on the planet, but they didn't need to know that right away.

Recruiting is one of the only parts of the Marines where you get to have a say in where you are sent, rather than taking an order to be sent to another part of the world. I started off in San Diego at the recruitment school. The little boy from Ohio, who would always sit at the front and ask the teacher constant questions, was a memory. As a shy person and an introvert, it was a tough process, because it was entirely public speaking and communication. It was also my first time living in a big city alone, with no one like my sister to hold my hand, so it was an eye-opener. Every single day we had to get up and give a speech for thirty minutes, about whatever topic the instructor came up with, and you had to know everything about every Marine role, in detail. A required part of the course was the anger speech, where you would spend forty-five minutes building up your emotions until you were screaming and tossing chairs in the classroom, before you had to calm yourself down again. We were constantly being evaluated, and I didn't think I had what it took, but by the end of the course, I had gotten the hang of it, and was ready to try and sign up as many recruits as possible.

What I remember most about the school was that it was a crash course in alcohol and hangovers. I was twenty-one and my roommate was born in Tijuana, so every weekend we would drive fifteen minutes to cross the Mexican border and party in his hometown. There were many girls, which didn't matter because I was still single, and plenty of booze. We would get back on a Monday morning with extreme hangovers, and would be asked to do fitness tests that I would barely pass.

After graduating, I had to select where I wanted to be sent to work as a recruiter. The dream was Hawaii, Florida, or close to home in Ohio. I put all three options down, hoping I would have the chance of getting one, but I got word from the school that a Sergeant Major had put in a request to send me to a specific location, meaning he had chosen me for a specific assignment. Then they told me it was Pittsburgh. "What the hell is this?" I asked, completely dumbstruck and angry. I was told that Medina—the station I was recruited out of in Ohio—was at 120 percent capacity for staff and didn't need any more, and Florida was out of the question because I was white, and didn't speak Spanish like a lot of the potential recruits walking into the office. I didn't get to find out why Hawaii was taken off the list, but I was bound for Pennsylvania, so at least I only had a four-hour drive back to see my family. The office was in Johnstown, a thirty-minute drive to Shanksville, where United Flight 93 went down on 9/11. I had never been to New York, and a visit to the crash site brought back all the memories of the carnage and death from that day, and reminded me why I was still serving.

I was young to be a recruiter, but when it came to combat I was more experienced than the rest of my crew, who hadn't been overseas. I met my senior officer, and he gave me my first orders straight away: "Across the street is a mall. You have forty-five minutes, and you are going to introduce yourself to everyone who works in each of the stores."

I walked out in uniform. All the shoppers were carrying their bags and walking with their kids, looking at my haircut. They seemed to give me a wide berth when I passed them. It was almost as disconcerting as a patrol in Kabul. I approached every clerk and cashier in the coffee shops, in the shoe stores, and in all the kiosks, shook their hands, and said: "Hello, I'm Sergeant Bee and I am the new Marine recruiter."

Some of them smiled awkwardly and said "hi" back, but others would stay silent, or just nod and go back to work. I have never been someone who enjoys small talk, so each interaction was as painful as the last. I kept going, and made my way to the food court. I headed towards the jewelry stores, and that's when I saw a blonde woman standing behind one of the counters, who made me stop in my tracks. I kept looking through the window at her, and watched as she looked out at customers and laid out necklaces in front of her. She was gorgeous. I knew this store was definitely one place I had to stop in and show my face. I combed back what little hair I had with my hand, straightened my collar up, and made sure my shirt was completely clean. I didn't want her to notice even a speck of food or a stain. I coughed, stood up straight, and—trying my best to look casual in military attire—walked inside. She locked eyes with me as soon as I walked in, and her expression didn't change one bit. To her, I was just like every other customer. I kept moving forward and slowly made my way to the counter, and when I arrived, she didn't seem the least bit interested.

I held out my palm, which was sweating by that point, and said, in what I thought was my coolest, most manly voice: "I'm Sergeant Bee, nice to meet you. I am the new Marine recruiter."

She looked at my hand for a second and then turned her eyes back to me.

"Okay. I'm Bobbie," she said, and just walked away as if nothing had happened. Bobbie had no interest in anything I had to say. I felt ridiculous. I stood there for a moment, stunned and embarrassed, and left as quickly as I could. I had lost the first battle with a humiliating result, but I knew I would be back. I would see her on lunch breaks and would bump into her walking around, so I knew I would get a second shot at some point. I was a strapping Marine who had been to war—how could she turn me down? I had been taught to be able to sell anything at recruiter school, so why couldn't I sell myself, even if she was way out of my league?

Meanwhile, the recruitment job was by far the worst job I had ever had in my life, and I quickly started regretting my decision to take it on. My shift would start at 6 a.m., and it wouldn't finish until I had set up three interviews and had three appointments. Sign-up quotas were essential, so I had to try to meet my goals and stick to them. Some days, I would get three interviews during the first two hours and could relax the rest of the day, but other times I would be cruising around gas stations at 1 a.m., trying to track down anyone who would come into the office and consider becoming a grunt. I would beg them for an interview just so I could go home. But I got to go back to a bed in a condo every night and if I finished before 11 p.m I could spend the nights going out to bars. I could take trips on the rare weekends I got off. It was as close to a normal life as you could get while you were in the Marines. My team was tight, and we spent all day and most nights together. We would hit dollar-beer nights and the local clubs **hard**, when we clocked off.

I would go to a kid's house or invite them to the office for a two-hour sales pitch, like the one I had received just three years earlier. I would be as aggressive as I could, to see if they could withstand the pressure. On Sundays, I would drive those who wanted to take the next steps to the MEPS (Military Enlistment Processing Center), to put them through every doctor's test imaginable. I wanted to make sure every kid was healthy enough to get in, but also warned them to be very careful with what they put down in their histories, to save themselves a mountain of paperwork. I didn't want to do anything illegal, but I told them: "If you broke your arm when you were six years old, keep your mouth shut. You don't want the doctors to have to track down twenty pages of medical reports from ten years ago. The answers are 'No,' 'Never,' and 'Not that I am aware of.'"

Most of the recruits stuck in my memory, even though we went through each process so quickly. Once we signed them up, the focus was getting them in shape for boot camp and making sure they graduated; otherwise the recruiting team wouldn't get any credit. The whole job was about numbers. You could be the best Marine on the planet, but if you didn't get enough contracts signed, you were looked at as a piece of shit by senior officers. And the kids you approached to try and recruit would sometimes treat you like a piece of dirt on their shoes. I would go up to them with a smile, shake their hands, and say: "Hey, do you want to join the Marines?"

"Go fuck yourself," the little brats would respond and laugh at me, to the point where I wanted to throw them off the second deck of the mall. I knew there were thousands of reasons not to want to join, but their lack of respect filled me with rage, because I knew my men on the other side of the world were sacrificing everything. We were protecting these kids and trying to make sure our nation wasn't attacked again, and some Marines and sailors were dying for it.

I tried to keep my spirits up by sticking with my crew, hitting the bars whenever I could, and paying Bobbie visits. I found any excuse I could to go near her jewelry store on break, and would sit and eat my lunch outside her window without looking at her, trying to play it cool. There were only a couple of bars and clubs in town, the mall was small, and we had mutual friends, so we would end up hanging out at the same places, night after night. At first she wasn't interested, but I kept trying. One of my buddies was dating one of Bobbie's friends, so he would sometimes bring me along, knowing that I was dead set on dating her. On a night where none of the bands we liked were playing in the clubs, or when the drinks weren't discounted at one of the bars, we decided to hang at a house and watch a movie. I walked in the door and looked at Bobbie's face, and her eyes rolled. She didn't know I was coming, and I could see by the look in her eyes that she was dreading spending the night with this idiot Marine, who she was already annoyed with. But when our friends went to bed, Bobbie and I stayed up and talked all night. My affection for her only grew stronger when I finally left in the morning, and I hoped that she was starting to feel the same way. I needed more nights when nothing was going on in Johnstown, so I had an excuse to just sit and talk to her, for hours and hours without interruption.

She was the hardest girl to get in the mall, and my boss knew I liked her, so he offered me a wager that he thought could help me in my pursuit. He was going out for lunch and told me: "If you can get a date with her by the time I get back, I will set up all your appointments with recruits for a week. If you can't, you will set up all the appointments for the rest of the team."

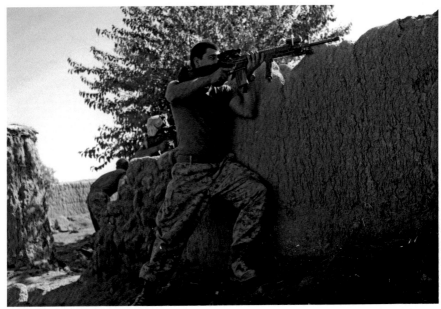

Preparing to fire back at a Taliban sniper in Garmsir, Helmand Province, in May 2008. *Photo courtesy of Goran Tomasevic and Reuters.*

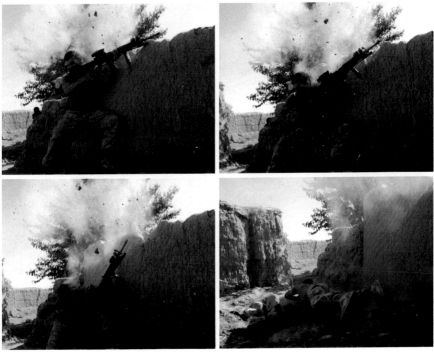

The close call with the Taliban sniper round in Garmsir, Helmand Province, in May 2008, captured by Reuters photographer Goran Tomasevic.

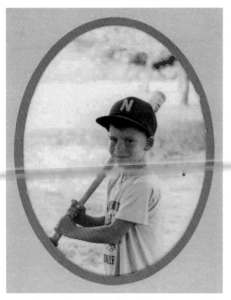

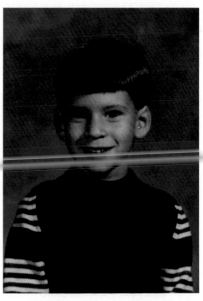

Me playing baseball for Northwestern in Ohio in 1987

Me at elementary school in Ohio in 1987

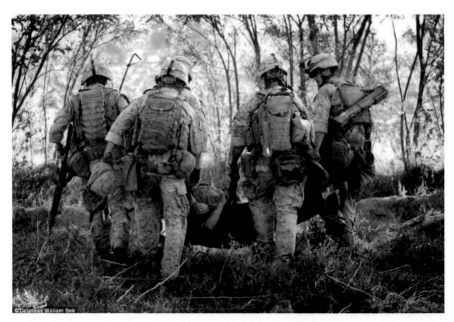

Marines carry me away from the IED blast in Marjah, Helmand Province, 2010, on the last day of combat of my career.

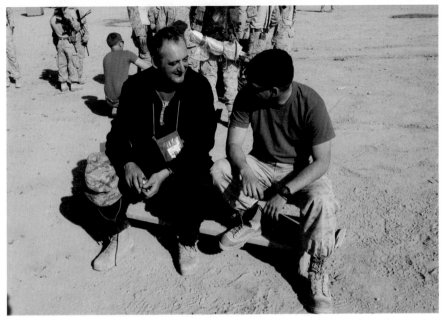

Reunited with Goran Tomasevic in Marjah, Helmand Province, before the major combat operation in 2010.

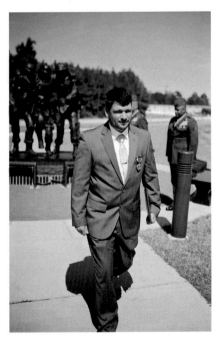

Receiving the Purple Heart in 2016 after years of Bobbie's paperwork on my traumatic brain injuries. *Photo courtesy of Chrissie Kirk.*

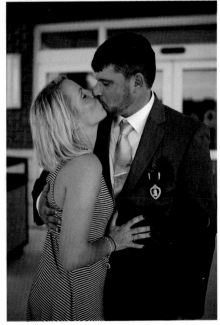

Bobbie and I during the Purple Heart ceremony in 2016. *Photo courtesy of Chrissie Kirk.*

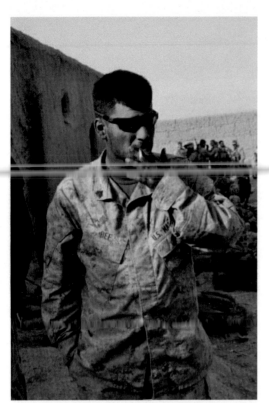

Me in Marjah during a break in combat operations in 2010.

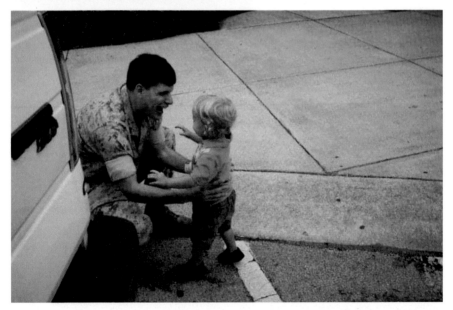

Reunited with Ethan at Camp Lejeune, North Carolina, after returning from treatment for my injuries in Landsthul, Germany, in 2010.

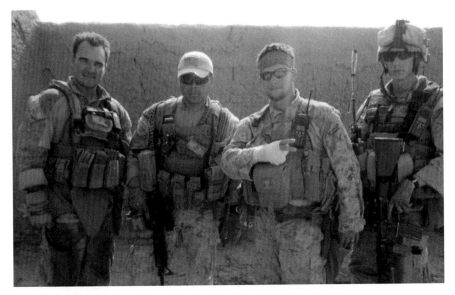

Butler, Matt, Me, Weckman in Marjah, Helmand Province, in April 2010.

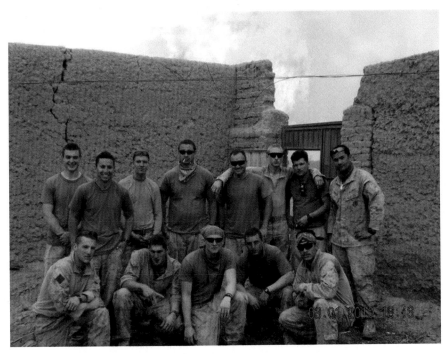

(Left to right) 1st row: LCpl Hoelle, LCpl Tatum, Doc Gray, LCpl Berstein, LCpl Gonzalez
2nd row: LCpl Johnston, Cpl Alires, LCpl Dow, Cpl Ponce, Cpl Butler, LCpl Weckman,
Sgt Bee, Cpl Winston.

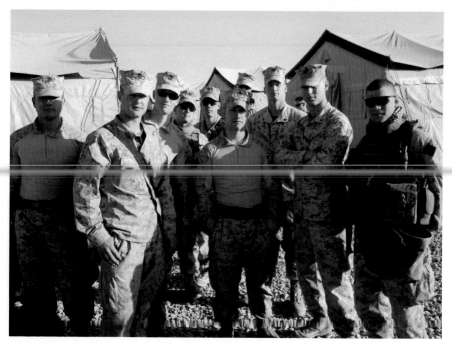

(Left to right) LCpl Winston, LCpl Bozanich, LCpl Dykstra, LCpl Connel, LCpl Bremer, Cpl Campbell, Cpl Achey, LCpl Wycka, Sgt Bee 3rd Squad 4th Platoon Alpha co 1/6 in Garmsir, Helmand Province, 2008.

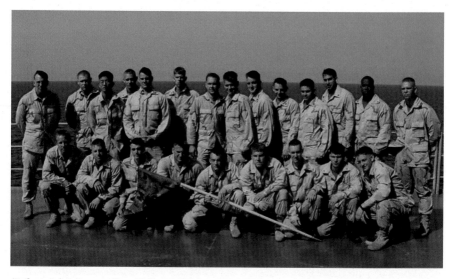

(Left to right) 1st row: Doc Hall, LCpl Tobin, LCpl Kirby, LCpl Wyland, LCpl Smith, LCpl Rizzo, L Cpl Hubbard, LCpl Bee, LCpl Morris 2nd row: Lt Himes, LCpl Spaulding, LCpl DeCamp, Cpl Davis, Cpl Clark, LCpl Harris, LCpl Pazgan, LCpl Schuster, Cpl Eggers, Cpl Larson, Sgt Stover, Cpl Shearer, Cpl Messiah, Sgt Morris 2nd Platoon Lima co 3/6.

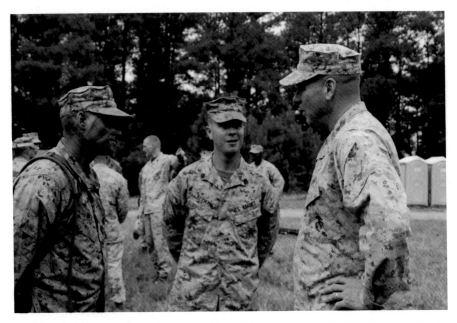

Me, Staff Sergeant Kerman and Brigadier General Simmons at the Field Medical Battalion in Florida in 2012.

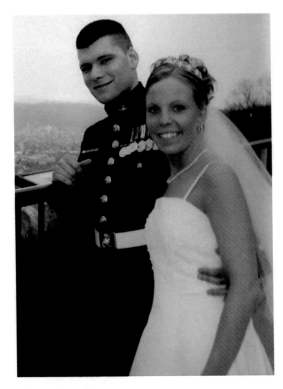

My wedding day with Bobbie in Pennsylvania on April 1, 2006, during my deployment as a recruiter.

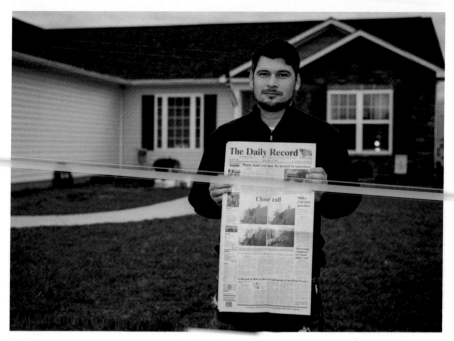

Holding a newspaper front page with "The Shot" photo at my home in Jacksonville, North Carolina, in 2015. *Photo courtesy of Nick Pironio from DailyMail.com.*

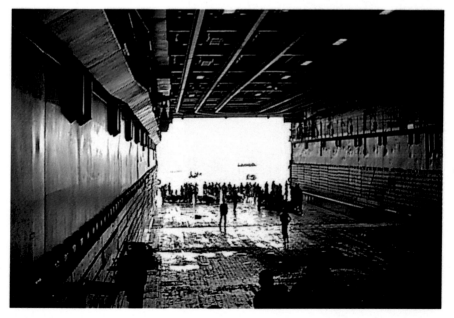

Zodiak Boat recovery USS Shreveport 2001.

During one of my interviews, I saw her walking past my window and I told the kid I would be back in a minute. I ran outside just so I could talk to her, and ten minutes later I had forgotten I was in the middle of an application. Somehow, I had managed to grow on her, and—during my boss's lunch break that day—I succeeded in asking her out. We started dating. A month later was the Marine's birthday ball, at a casino in West Virginia. (On November 10th every year, Marines around the globe celebrate the day the Corps was created—in 1775, at a bar called the Tun Tavern in Philadelphia. From there, they started their first drive for recruits during the American Revolution.) It was a huge party and I had only been with Bobbie for a few weeks, so I didn't know if she wanted to go with me. Little did I know she had already found out about it, when she invited me to a dress shop to watch her try on clothes. She stepped out of the dressing room with her first outfit on and said: "So, is this what I am wearing to the ball?" She had made herself my plus-one, and I wasn't going to say no.

For the next two years, Bobbie and the friends on my team were my only source of happiness. I quickly stopped caring about recruiting numbers, even though in my second year I was runner-up in the competition for the most signed contracts. The long days, and endless appointments with teenage boys who looked down their noses at you, were soul-destroying, and I was close to giving up. I had no motivation left and wasn't sure where the job was taking me. The moment I really lost it was when my grandma died. My relationship with my family was still up and down, and she was part of a tumultuous childhood, but it still hurt me. I wanted to go to her funeral, so I needed to take time off. But my boss—a new guy—said no, and told me I had to get another contract. When I was denied leave, I also found out a guy had been promoted in front of me, even though I had signed more recruits, so I trashed my office and flipped my desk. I still had a year to go and I had to try and stay the course.

My schedule was even an issue when Bobbie and I decided to get married, after just a year of dating. We were in love, and I was spending all the free time I had with her, so all we needed to do was find a day when I could escape work, and tie the knot. I was gung-ho about a huge wedding and party any Marine would be proud of, wearing my full dress blues with the sword at the ceremony. Bobbie initially wanted to elope, but she caved to my nagging about having a big celebration. She said she wanted a spring wedding, and found out the church we both wanted to get married in—down the road from the mall—had an opening on Saturday, April 1. The start of the month was when there was less pressure to meet recruitment numbers and try to meet deadlines. The date was set, our families and friends came into town, and we were ready for a party. The night before the wedding, I was working late as usual when I realized I still had to pick up my dress blues from the dry cleaner's—I didn't have anything else to wear. But the cleaner's was closed and just one member of staff was left. Luckily, I managed to force my way in with one of the groomsmen, demanding they hand my dress blues over. They did, and we went back to my condo for the night. Bobbie and I lived in the condo together, but she wasn't there because we wanted to keep up the tradition of staying apart the night before the wedding, so she was staying with her family and best friend from California.

The next morning, I woke up at my condo alongside my groomsmen and got changed into my dress blues. I was ready to marry the girl I'd fallen for at the mall, who had picked me up during one of the most frustrating times of my life. I was excited for a day not thinking about appointments, recruitment numbers, my boss, or any of the asshole kids who mocked me when I asked if they wanted to join the military. I was free for a day, or so I thought.

The phone started ringing. It could have been someone asking to pick something up or ask directions to the church, but no—it was my office saying I had to come in and fix something.

"On the most important day of my life? Are you fucking serious?"

"We'll have you back for the ceremony, don't worry," the officer said on the other end of the line. I reluctantly took off my dress blues and put my uniform back on. I drove back to the office and quickly finished fixing whatever they had done wrong, and I still had a few hours to spare until the wedding. Bobbie was running around stressed, so I decided it was best not to tell her I had gone back to work.

We were still fixing our uniforms when we drove up to the church and screeched to a stop in front of everyone walking up the steps to go inside. All that mattered was I was there in one piece with my shoes shined, my hat on straight, and my collar as high as the truest jarhead. That's what I wanted for my wedding, and it's all I wanted for Bobbie. My life had changed so much in the year since I had walked into her jewelry store and she had rejected me on the spot. I always wondered how a girl who was just five-foot-one could make such an enormous impact, and how she could become a line of defense for someone who could be away for months on end. I had fallen in love with her harder than I ever could have imagined, and as I saw her walking down the aisle in her beautiful dress, arm in arm with her dad, all I could do was stare in amazement. I cried when I saw her. We weren't really an emotional couple and would share more laughs than tears, but that day I struggled to hold it together. She looked so beautiful I couldn't help myself, so when she arrived at the altar and I pulled the veil off of her face, I whispered to her: "You look so hot."

I forgot we had microphones on, and everyone in the pews started giggling. It was April Fool's Day after all, and there were still some people who thought the wedding was a joke.

Many tears were shed that day, even by some of the Marines standing beside me, and we partied that night as hard as we had done since we first met in Johnstown. We had disposable cameras instead of a professional photographer, Bobbie's dad's country band played the reception, and many shots of tequila were downed. That day was one of the few—in the first twenty-two years of my life—that I made the happiest memories, that would take me through some of the darkest moments to come, and could bring a smile to my face in some of the ugliest places on earth.

I didn't plan a honeymoon because I didn't know how much time I was going to get off. Knowing how my bosses had reacted to news of my step-grandmother's funeral, I didn't think I would get any. So the night after we got married, Bobbie and I decided to rent a car and drive to New York for three days in Manhattan, before I had to be back in the office. As we made our way through the city streets, the crowds of people, the noise, and the traffic terrified me. I had never been in a place that could even compare to New York's size and utter chaos. so I spent most of the time grabbing onto Bobbie's arm. We arrived on Monday night, and wanted to get on camera at NBC's *Today Show*, so we applied for a place at Rockefeller Plaza for the following morning. I had never been anywhere like New York. It was something we had always talked about doing, and it would have been perfect less than forty-eight hours after we walked down the aisle. But after we registered and made our placards. I stopped at a food cart on one of the street corners for a hot dog, and got food poisoning. The first time I ever went to a Starbucks in my life was to vomit in the toilet. I thanked God that—even back then—there was one on every street corner. I spent the rest of the night in the hotel being violently sick, and thought to myself: "This is a great way to start our marriage. This can't be a good sign, or it can only go up from here."

After spending the night crouched over the toilet of our Midtown hotel room, I managed to drag myself back out and back to Rockefeller Plaza, to get on TV. We got on screen for a few seconds, and cheered up everyone who was recording it on their VCRs back home, before we got a picture with Al Roker.

We then did what everyone should do their first time in New York: we went the Statue of Liberty, attended our first Broadway show (*Beauty and the Beast*—Bobbie's choice, despite my protests), visited a comedy club, got lost in Macy's and ended up walking around for hours, and then got so drunk we almost missed our subway stop on the way back to our hotel.

We also decided to go to Ground Zero. In 2005, there was no memorial or buildings. It was still a building site with construction vehicles still moving the steel girders that remained, and investigators looking for anything that could identify the missing. Families of those who were still lost, and first responders, hung photos and messages on the chain-link fence surrounding the huge hole in the ground. Tourists just stopped and stood in silence, as they tried to come to terms with just how devastating that morning four years before had been. I broke down in tears. After three deployments it hit me hard—seeing the ruins for the first time—and all of my experiences started flooding back to me: the morning I watched the planes fly into the towers at Camp Lejeune, the beam on the deck of the first ship I was on in the Persian Gulf, the orphanage in Kabul, the first Taliban firefight, the lines of people greeting us along the road on our way back from the second tour. It reminded me again why I was a Marine and why I was helping fight the War on Terror. To see the pure emotion and the burning hole—caused by terrorists in the middle of a city that brings joy to so many, including Bobbie and I—was heartbreaking, and filled me with the rage I had felt so many times since I had signed up. It was the best honeymoon I could have asked for with my dream girl, and it made me realize more than ever where I needed to be.

My recruiting numbers started going down when I got back to Pennsylvania, with only nine months left in the assignment. I still went out and talked to kids and kept my head down, but my motivation had disappeared. What I realized about the job was that it was about the contracts you got, and nothing to do with the effort you put in for hours every day. If you were training and you couldn't hike for nine miles with your gear on, but you busted your ass to do it, you would get some credit. One of the only upsides to recruiting was that you got to pick where you went for your next deployment, but it only happened to those who were popular with command staff, Because of my performance over the last previous months, I wasn't given any favors.

I was told there wasn't a single spot for an infantry sergeant in Camp Pendleton, where I wanted to go; I had a choice of either Twentynine Palms, or with the 1st Battalion, 6th Marines at Camp Lejeune. Twentynine Palms was the sphincter of America: it smelled like shit and it was in the middle of the desert, hours away from any real civilization. There was no way in hell I was going back there, so I went with the 1st Battalion, 6th Marines in North Carolina, back to where my career had begun.

Bobbie moved with me to Jacksonville, and we had two weeks to try and find a house before I reported for duty. We were expecting to be assigned housing on Camp Lejeune straight away, but we were told there weren't any spaces because 75,000 more Marines had been added since I had been on recruiting duty. So, we hopped from hotel to hotel, and were on the phone with realtors day and night, trying to find a place to stay. We ended up getting a good house on what I considered the bad side of Jacksonville. It wasn't the best area to live, but it gave us a roof over our head, until one day when I was away from home—taking part in a field operation—a man was shot in the head and executed, three houses down. We managed to escape after a few months and got into housing on base.

I checked in with staff at the base and was assigned to Alpha company to do paperwork in the headquarters section. I hated every minute of it—I sucked at paperwork and my Sergeant made me miserable. For two months, I sat behind a desk, dotting i's and crossing t's, before I got into the squad leaders course, where I could get back to doing what I loved. I learned to fire mortars and artillery rounds and call for close air support, and I got back into shape after three years in Johnstown. In nine weeks, I developed more knowledge than I had ever had in my previous seven years in the Marines, and all the guys we were training with were at their peaks. They had been deployed and had been in heavy action—including the Battle of Ramadi, when Iraq was at its most vicious in 2006—so they knew what they were doing, but they had also lost a lot of guys.

It was 2008, and after the course had finished, we found out we would be heading to Afghanistan on what would be my fourth deployment. Since I'd left Kabul in 2003 Helmand Province had gotten more dangerous. The number of American casualties had been creeping up, firefights were getting more frequent, and the chances of you returning to the United States in one piece were getting slimmer. The Taliban had been forced out of the cities to the hills in the South, where they were still holding out and fighting—especially in

Kandahar Province where they were sending me—and Osama Bin Laden's location was still a mystery to the American government. It didn't look like the war would be ending any time soon, unlike a few years earlier when we had thought it would be over in a matter of weeks. I knew the next deployment was going to be intense, and I was convinced I wasn't going to get away with just one firefight and a couple of stray rounds.

My squad in Fourth Platoon was tighter than any other squad I had been in up to that point. I would have gatherings at my house and we would go out drinking together, while continuing to work towards the next trip. Then I found out Bobbie was pregnant. We had been married for two years and it wasn't a surprise, but realizing I would be away while she was carrying our first child was a punch in the gut. I was praying I would be back in time to see her give birth, but I knew it was out of my control. She was always there for me no matter what happened, and she was aware of the sacrifices she was making when she married me, but for me to not be there—for the one moment she needed me the most—was going to weigh on my mind constantly. Knowing I had her, and a bigger family to come back to, was more motivation I needed to make sure I didn't get killed. I wasn't nervous about the action; I was excited and I had supreme confidence in the men around me.

On the day we shipped out, Bobbie had an ultrasound to find out the sex of the baby. Normally the base is on lockdown that close to when you leave and no one is allowed off, but my sergeants made sure I could sneak out to get to the appointment. I made sure it was in the morning, because we were catching a bus to the airport and flying out that afternoon. I got in a car and got to the clinic in record time, to find out we were having a boy. That moment is incredible for any new parents, but for us the emotions were all over the place. We had a few minutes to cheer, cry, hug, and celebrate the news before I was in the car with her, heading back to base. Bobbie was trying to hold it together for me. She was tough as nails, so I knew she would handle it, but my heart was breaking, knowing I would be thousands of miles from her and would barely be able to speak to her. Then I was on the bus, and Bobbie was waving me off with her hand cradling her stomach. My hope was that I would be back in a few months to see her again, with our new son in her arms.

CHAPTER 8

I landed in Kyrgyzstan—one thousand miles northeast of Kabul—with the rest of the squad, after a short stop in Shannon, Ireland. The Central Asian country was very similar to our final destination: surrounded by mountains, landlocked, and like time had been standing still for decades. Until 1991, it was under control of the Soviet Union and the streets still had the signs to show it. Statues of Lenin stood outside eerie concrete apartment blocks, and there was a quiet that unnerved even me. I'd never seen anything like it. It was a ghost town—nothing like the ports in Italy and Spain, where we'd been able to drink wine and feast ourselves, before we touched down to start the deployment.

We were there to just wait, until we got called up to fly over the Hindu Kush mountains and into Helmand Province. My squad slept in a warehouse on an Air Force base, with five hundred other troops from other ISAF (International Security Assistance Force) countries. We were allowed two beers a night.

We also had very slow internet access, so I could keep in touch with Bobbie while she was going through her first stages of morning sickness and trying to deal with her pregnancy alone. But I was also pumped up and ready to fight, with some of the best guys in the business. Most of them had done tours in Iraq and had got chewed up pretty badly—with casualties and injuries during the bloodiest months in Ramadi—but I was the only one who had been to Kandahar. When we landed, it was unrecognizable. When I had been here before, I had sat in a hole for hours every day, and stared at the mountains outside a bombed-out base that was barely a few hangars and a couple of runways. Now, it was the command center for operations in southern Afghanistan, and there were thousands of members of ISAF forces and huge media operations. There was even a hockey rink, where members of the Stanley Cup team had played.

The Marines were stationed on the north side of the airfield, away from the rest of the U.S. forces, and we were the only ones allowed there. Our tents were three hundred yards away from the fence line where I had spent some of the most boring days of my life, and an hour away from the Green Bean coffee stand and Burger King, where we could enjoy a little slice of home comforts. A few years on from my first deployment, they were still clearing landmines from the surrounding area, and there was still a danger to us if one of them blew, but the entire base was a fortress in the middle of the desert, and a staging area for one of the biggest operations against the Taliban since the start of the war.

For the first few weeks, it was quiet. We would go out on patrol and train while the Army would fly in, hitting different areas in Helmand to establish a presence against the Taliban. We trained like I had done so many times before: putting on all our gear and packs, adding about a hundred pounds to our body mass, and doing laps around the airfield—in the heat during the day and when it was cold at night, so we could acclimatize. We would hit the shooting range and would train with the Army mortar teams, to give us the best chance possible of pushing the terrorists back. It was to get us ready to fly into Garmsir whenever we were needed. The district was a crucial supply route for the Taliban: it was made up of clusters of mud houses, irrigation canals that added an extra dimension to the kind of combat we could engage in, and a network of bazaars that all needed clearing. Most of the thousands of Afghans—living in the deeply impoverished corner of an already poverty-stricken country—had been told to leave by the insurgents, and the endless thunder of low-flying U.S. helicopters had scared the rest away. There were a few farmers left to help harvest the rest of the poppies for the opium trade, but many of the bulbs had already been scraped and the fields were barren. The psychological operations units were dropping pamphlets from helicopters, warning the natives to leave if they weren't Taliban, because anyone who was still around and was moving would be killed. The Taliban were also telling everyone to get out, because they wanted a standoff with the Americans. They were ready for a pure gunfight with nothing standing in their way. Tactically, it was a stupid move, because it meant everything else in the area was a potential target. I soon learned that it was going to be the largest helicopter assault since the Vietnam War, and Marines were telling the media that this was the operation to take control of Helmand Province. We were part of something huge, and I was excited.

In March 2008, a team flew up from Camp Dwyer—a base southwest of Garmsir where the British Royal Scots Guards and Gurkhas were stationed—to prepare for our first operation. The plan was a helicopter assault: drop in and set up a checkpoint, try to disrupt the Taliban supply lines, and set up our own transport line. Our senior officers told us we wouldn't be there for long, and to only bring a small D-pack—the size of a child's rucksack—with the bare essentials. They said the operation would only last a few weeks, but we still stuffed everything we could inside, and the helicopters could only take a certain amount of weight on board. I went from 160 pounds to around 250 pounds, with all the ammo I was cramming into every last space in the bag. The squad leaders warned us that we were going to use up most of our rounds trying to find these guys. I could barely move my arms because I had so many jackets on, and the platoon commanders started handing out mortar rounds to carry on us, because we didn't have the trucks to carry them. We ended up carrying them in our pockets, or strapping them to our legs and on our uniforms with duct tape. For the first three days after dropping us in the middle of enemy territory, we would be fighting ourselves out, until we had a supply column to bring in more ammunition and resources. It was insane how much equipment each man was carrying for what was supposed to be a short-term mission.

We then flew into Camp Bastion, another base controlled by the British at the time, to get ready to stage our assault. I was briefed; our squad would be on one of the first heli copters to land in the middle of the night, because we had experience and had built up a reputation for being one of the better-prepared groups of men, with clear fighting ability. We were given the objective to go into Garmsir and were ready for battle.

My squad was in the first wave of sixty helicopters to land in Indian Territory—in the middle of nowhere, in pitch black and eerie quiet. It was a textbook arrival straight out of training camp: everybody got off and watched as they flew out, to make way for the second group of arrivals. We had to wait twenty minutes for the next group to touch down, in a creepy nothingness I had never experienced in combat. In my first tour I was in a fighting hole, and in my second I was patrolling inside the confines of a heavily-guarded embassy, but in the middle of this field we had no cover, and any support had just flown away. We got on with our first field test: stop, listen, search, and smell, to see if there was anything out of the ordinary in our surroundings—but there was just dead silence. All you could hear were the boots of my men lightly treading the ground, as they scoured the night, looking for anything that might put us in danger.

My squad was tasked with clearing a building immediately outside the landing zone. The building glowed green through our night vision goggles as we approached in the darkness. Dykstra, our point man, suddenly called a halt and we all took a knee. Campbell went to check what was going on, when the silence was broken by a beep on my radio.

"Sergeant Bee, can I get you up here," Campbell said to me.

"Dude, is it something we can push through? We've got to clear this building before the next wave gets here." I replied. We were trying to be ninjas and get to cover without any detection. Most of the civilians had left the area, but we still didn't know if any Taliban were in the area. One of their best combat skills was hiding, and in a firefight you would rarely see one of them up close. Some Marines never even saw a member of the Taliban in the flesh, during their tours. Every second we took getting to the building and breaching it gave more time to the enemy to wake up, grab their gear and take up a position.

"There is a bear up here," Campbell said back. I stopped in my tracks and stared at the radio, confused as hell. There was no way a bear was roaming the middle of the southern Afghanistan countryside. So I snuck up to the front of our formation to see what was going on, and saw a giant, furry thing that looked like a monster on the ground. It was the first time I had ever seen one of the giant Caucasian shepherds the Afghans used to protect their homes and flocks, from people and wolves. It must have been about two hundred pounds and bigger than most of the men in my team. Campbell and I just stared in awe for a few seconds at the monster sleeping in front of us, then stepped over it and kept moving. None of us liked the idea of shooting a dog; we'd much rather shoot a Taliban. The fact was, though, one of those beasts could tear a Marine up if they came at us.

We got to the building and it was full of men, women, and children. Some of the locals had stayed behind to harvest the last of the poppy crop, but we didn't know where they were going to show up and how they would react to us. Our translator—who wanted us to call him John, for John Rambo—started talking to the men in the group, while the women and the kids were taken into another room inside. The locals were weirdly calm, considering a group of American men armed to the teeth and covered in camouflage paint had just barged in at three o'clock in the morning.

The interpreter—our "terp,"—told them not to worry, that we weren't going to hurt them and would pay for anything we damaged, but they needed to get the hell out of the building and to safety as soon as possible. This was going to be our COC (the Combat Operations Center or command post)—hundreds more Marines, who the Taliban were trying to hunt down, would be arriving in the next few minutes. While we waited for Alpha and Bravo companies to fly in, we started setting up M18 Claymore mines around the compound, to help initiate an ambush if the enemy tried an attack, and then got ready to leave at first light.

I got a few hours' sleep head-to-toe with my squad members, wearing most of our gear, and woke up to it already being 100 degrees and 99 percent humidity outside. It was disgusting. A journalist in his fifties, who embedded with us, had already tapped out and said he couldn't carry on. We were relieved, because he was an extra weight we wouldn't have to carry.

We packed up, left the compound, and started walking, with the unforgiving sun and heat bearing down on us with every step. My squad hadn't even moved a mile when we got our first contact. It was the first time I had been under fire since Kandahar. A shot cracked in between all of us. I relied on muscle memory and hit the ground straight away. My point man just face-planted on the ground because he was exhausted.

"Contact!" everyone started screaming, and I tried to find out where the round was coming from. I looked up from the ground, left and right, to see if I could spot anything. Was it

Taliban or a farmer warning us to get off his land? After a few seconds I got up, and our squad ran to get in line—a formation we had been trained to use when we were under fire. But nothing came after the first round. I stood there and looked at my guys scouring the area, looking for the gunman—but nothing. We waited a minute for the adrenaline to subside, and for everyone to calm down. It could have been anything, but we decided it was fine to advance. After a few more seconds, the rounds started flying again. We were under heavy fire. I knew they weren't close, and we couldn't see them, but it was constant and it seemed they were shooting and moving to try and outflank us. We then opened up and started going to town by spraying fire all the way around us. The 3rd Regiment was also heavily engaged nearby, so they set up a blocking position to stop the Taliban from reaching us, which meant we could get to our next building for some cover. It wasn't much, but I knew—after just a few hours in Garmsir— that this would be different, that it would be more intense and heated than what I had expected. We were bringing it to the Taliban, but they were determined to stand their ground, and protect the poppy fields that provided most of the financial backing for their whole militant operation.

In the first six or seven hours, we had only advanced three miles because of the heat, the weight of our gear, and the fire coming at us. We had only cleared six or seven buildings, but we found a decent position to hole up in for the night. We had to check each house, mud hut, bazaar, or compound we found, to make sure there were no Taliban inside and to tell the civilians to leave. We kicked down doors as we slowly made our way across farmland, in the unforgiving Afghan summer. Everyone was exhausted and desperate for a place to lay their heads for a few hours' rest, before we had to do it all again.

My squad spotted a house to take over for the night, approached, knocked down the door, and walked in. I explored room by room, and determined that the man who lived there had already fled but had left his animals behind, including the rabbits who were living in his cooking area, where the pots and pans would have normally been. The farmers in Southern Helmand had an unusually close relationship with their animals, especially during the winter when temperatures would drop below zero, and they would sometimes sleep with them for warmth. I was shocked people could live like that, but it's what happens when millions in your country are driven to poverty. I didn't get much sleep, because a rooster kept crowing every hour throughout the night.

So I woke up and kept busy by looking around the compound. I found a locked door behind a wall that was a lot bigger than the others, that I hadn't checked. I kicked it in, and I saw dozens of jugs stacked inside a small room the size of a closet, and then I caught the smell of ammonia. I thought, *This can't be good.* I called Campbell, my team leader, and told him to come over so he could check it out. He told me it was ammonium nitrate, and there were charges inside with the canisters. There must have been seventy pounds of explosives inside. My men had been sleeping just a few feet away from explosives, and none of us had a clue. If I hadn't looked behind the wall, something could have caused the charges to go off. I could have had blood of the Marines on my hands. I could have been dead.

We made a few more calls, and found out that the house we had chosen for cover had been tagged as an IED production facility. It was bad juju, and we needed to do something about it, to make sure the Taliban couldn't return and use the explosives on western troops.

Campbell said, "We need to get rid of this shit. I have a bunch of cratering charges and explosives. We can use them." We got everyone out, and chased the rabbits and some chickens from inside the house to make sure they weren't in the blast zone. At that point, we had a higher regard for the sanctity of livestock than we did for the Taliban: there wasn't any need for the animals to die. We laid down eighty pounds of explosives and blew up the house and all of the liquids inside. The blast and the cloud of smoke were enormous, and there was nothing left but a hole in the ground.

We kept pushing on as if nothing had happened: clearing buildings, taking the odd round while we were moving, and trying to flush out the militants, before reaching a building overlooking the MEU (Marine expeditionary unit) objective the next day. We hunkered down in position, just waiting to hit our target, listening to little blackbirds chirping on the walls around us. (I started calling them "overhere" birds when I was on post, because their calls sounded like they were saying "over here, over here.")

Then the first signs of the fight started, and I got to experience a member of the Taliban in person for the first time. We were sitting and watching our target, when three men on a dirt bike rode up and stopped just a few meters away right in front of us. We were inside, with three belt-fed M240 machine guns trained on them. We didn't know if they were suicide bombers, or had no idea we were in the building and happened to stop by pure chance. But one of them had an AK-47, and when he raised it slightly that was it—everyone on the line opened up with their machine guns and their weapons, and the three of them weren't there for very long. I fired my rifle and hit him in the chest. They were all down, and the AK and the bike were left just lying on the ground, with a cloud of dust where the barrage of rounds had dug into the ground. It was the first kill for me, and the first for about thirteen others as well. It was exciting because the Taliban always fought from buildings or hid in the hills, and this was the first time we had them up close and got our shot. We moved the bodies, and for the next few hours we watched as other men would try and pick up the bike and the gun, and meet the same fate.

In the compound I found what felt like a bean bag under a rug, that I could use to sit on. It was comfy and the closest thing to a chair I could get my hands on. I thought the homeowners must have left it behind, so I used it to my advantage. On the first night I had the best night sleep I'd ever had during my deployments. When I wasn't sleeping, I would use it to rest my head in-between fights, because we had gotten used to taking a nap while bullets were flying. On the second day, the battalion commander came down, and brought with him a member of law enforcement—similar to an ATF or DEA agent—who dealt with criminal investigation and matters among the men while we were on the ground. He was the drug expert in a region where poppy seeds covered almost every field.

I was bullshitting to my squad, sitting on my self-made chair and pillow, when he came up to me and started laughing. "Do you know how much your chair is worth?" he asked me.

Very confused, I responded, "What the hell are you talking about? I just found it lying around."

He said, "That chair could be worth up to eleven million dollars."

I had no idea what he was talking about and started patting the bean bag. Then it dawned on me.

"That's heroin," he said. There must have been almost seventy pounds in the bag, with a street value of at least seven million dollars. He took it away, and I lost my chair.

We were in the position for a few more days on rotation: we were on post for four hours, then would rest for eight hours where we weren't allowed to fight. We would sleep in a room that wasn't much bigger than seven by twelve feet, with an entire squad and their weapons and gear, with fights going on just a few yards away. When we were on post, we shot across a river to the compound we were trying to take over, and we realized we were going to have to fight our way there. The gunfights were like clockwork, with one in the morning and one after calls to prayer.

During one of the fights, I had eyes on where the shots were coming from, but they were too far away to engage with our rifles, and there were other men to the right of the building we were trying to hit. I was crouched behind sandbags, watching the men in front of me aiming in the wrong place. We never left our compound to do anything, because every time you did, you were under fire almost immediately. It wasn't safe; in the compound we had enough cover to protect us when we needed to fire. But like a dumbass—without any thought of what I was doing, and not thinking of using the radio—I jumped over the barrier and jogged over with no cover and in open fire. I leaned down to one of the men and said, "You need to fire a little to the right with a bit more power."

The guy looked up at me like I was crazy and said, "Are you alright? What are you doing?"

"No, I'm fine," I said, and told them to pick up the Bushmaster twenty-five-millimeter cannon and open up on the building. I turned around and started jogging back to the compound without a care in the world, while my guys were waving at me to hurry up, from behind the sandbags. I dove back over the top, and one of the guys smacked me on the head and said, "What the hell were you thinking?"

"What? Their shooting was off by 160 yards. I had to tell them."

"Look at this," he said, and showed me a screen and a video someone had just taken of me. You could see me running like an idiot, waving to the guys in the compound, with rounds skipping past my legs, and puffs of dirt where the bullets were hitting the ground.

"Ah, so that's why everyone was shouting at me," I said, still not caring too much about what had happened. I still don't know whether I risked my life like that to get a message to my guys that they were shooting at the wrong target, or simply out of the boredom from being in that building for hours on end. Maybe I wanted to escape for just a second. It didn't even cross my mind that the Taliban would see me and start shooting.

The fighting was kinetic and constant. The Taliban would fire RPGs at least three times an hour, but they didn't know how to pull off the safety pins on the rocket heads, that stopped them from exploding. So the RPGs would smack the mud wall

example for the rest of the young grunts being shot at, while they were hunkered down next to the white tree. I decided to draw some fire.

I put my compass in my hand, picked up my knife, and ran into the middle of the poppy field. The rounds kept going off around me as I sprinted with my head down, and I was thinking to myself, *Where the fuck are these guys?* I then hit the ground and looked into the night, to try and get my bearings. It was dumb luck. I looked up for a second and spotted a muzzle flash at the end of the field. Now I knew where they were shooting from. I turned back, ran as quickly as my exhausted legs would carry me, and dove back behind the building to tell the rest of my squad where to aim. I was then able to get hold of a lieutenant, and call in a fire mission to take them out. I was awarded my first Navy Achievement Medal for running into the middle of a Taliban firefight. I thought I was being brave, but my squad thought I was plain stupid. If my wife Bobbie had known what I had done, she would have thought the same, considering we had a baby on the way, and I had a family to still provide for. My impulses always got the better of me; it would just be a couple of days until I found out that they could result in me paying the ultimate price, because after that night, we were onto the building that would forever etch my name in Marine history, in both a good and a bad way.

CHAPTER 9

Until that point in my third tour, no one close to me had been killed. Aside from a few close calls and rounds landing six or seven inches from our heads, we were all alive. There were some bruised egos, cuts and scrapes, and nights where we were so exhausted we didn't know how we would wake up for the next firefight. But we were in one piece.

One night, while crossing a metal beam over an irrigation canal, on a move to our next building, I fell into the water with my full gear and couldn't get back to the surface. A lance corporal had to pull me out. I was dead weight at the bottom and couldn't get out, and I probably would have stayed there if he hadn't dove in to save me. Once again, me being a sheer dumbass had put me at risk of death.

Before we were assigned another objective and more buildings to hit, I was told our squad would be picking up a journalist to embed with us. I didn't have high opinions of reporters following us around at the time, and only saw them as something that would slow us down. Only a few weeks before, a correspondent had decided to break off after eighteen hours because he couldn't stand the heat. I wasn't looking forward to meeting the new guy and he was going to have to do a lot to gain the respect of my men. We were patrolling to the command post to pick him up and everything seemed normal, when I suddenly got a call saying, "Bee, stop your patrol right now." We all dropped and took a knee, to wait and see what was going on. The COC rarely interrupted a patrol, so my heart started racing a little quicker. A few seconds went by and there was nothing but my squad on alert. Then, I heard on the radio: "Hey, you're good to keep going." Intelligence had discovered there was a Taliban sniper in the area targeting U.S. patrols, and they had intercepted communications with his commander. It was a bad omen, but we got the all clear, and carried on to pick up our embed.

Goran Tomasevic was a Serbian photographer who had been working for Reuters—the biggest news agency in the world—since 1996. He had seen more conflict than most Marines, having been on the ground following the break-up of Yugoslavia, and had covered the surge in violence in Iraq under Saddam Hussein.

At first, he looked like any other photographer with his PRESS flak jacket on, but his first gesture made sure he stood out from the rest. As I approached him to introduce myself, he reached into his bag and pulled out a container of Marlboro

Red cigarettes, and started handing them out to the squad. They were rare in Afghanistan and were usually sold by locals at a huge markup, because they had stolen them or picked them up when they had fallen off the back of a truck. The cigarettes made and sold in Afghanistan were dry as hell— like putting your mouth around a Humvee exhaust. When we saw the Reds with labels showing they were from the United States, we could have got down on our knees and worshipped Goran. Most of us had run out of smokes or chewing tobacco because our packs were so small and there was barely any room to store extras, so his gift cemented him as part of the team, and he knew it. We picked him up and moved on to the next target in Garmsir.

It was a small village, with two compounds facing each other and a poppy field to the east. The building we moved into was sat lower than two others surrounding it, so the Taliban could see us and we couldn't see behind their walls. We weren't receiving much fire at first. There were firefights going on around us, but none of the fire was directed our way. When I was on post, I thought someone kept shooting a mortar a few yards away from me and tried to figure out what the hell was going on. That's when I discovered the snipers were using fifty-caliber bullets the size of hot dogs which would break the sound barrier as they flew in front of our position.

The day came and went without much else happening, and that night I sat by my radio in the pitch black, staring into the void. I put on my night vision goggles at one point, and all I could see were the bugs crawling in the thatched roof above me, then some sort of insect with huge legs walked across my face and I let out a high-pitched scream. I managed to get a few hours of sleep until I was back on post the following morning.

I woke up to more frequent gunfire aimed at our compound, but it still wasn't enough to put us at any real risk, so I decided to wash some of my clothes before our shifts changed over and I was back on rest. I probably should have waited.

Doing laundry on an operation was like being back in the 1700s, when women and children scrubbed clothes on rocks to try and get them clean, and we would get so desperate for water we would use mud. Luckily, I was using a bar of soap I found while clearing out a bazaar and a rusty bucket with holes in the bottom, that kept having to be refilled. I'd used three pairs of underwear on rotation for all of our excursions and to sleep in, and the sweat had pretty much rotted them through. My socks were so crusty, I could stand them up when I put them on the floor. If only Bobbie could have seen me. I was sitting there, rinsing my filthy, worn-through garments, when I heard the first shot, and it was close. That's when I picked up my rifle, without my Kevlar or helmet on, and rushed to the wall to take position to try and find out where the sniper was firing from. The Taliban would only engage with us between three hundred and six hundred yards, because that was where their weapons—handed down from the Soviet Union—would be most effective, but a round getting that close to one of my guys meant that the marksman—with his hand on the trigger—was taking his time and knew what he was doing. Goran crouched beside me as I trained my sight to the south and the compound looking into ours. It was an advantageous position because the Taliban marksman was looking down on us. I turned to a mud hut, saw some movement behind a pile of laundry, and that's when everything turned to black.

It was an explosion just a few inches away from my head, and the loudest sound I had ever heard in my life. I could feel the impact reverberating, and it seemed like my brain was bouncing off the insides of my skull. I couldn't hear and I couldn't see. I felt myself slowly falling backwards towards the dirt hole I had just crawled out of. It seemed like time had stopped.

I still wasn't sure what had happened, but I couldn't move my arms to brace myself for the impact, as my body crumpled towards the ground. I landed on my back with a thud and my head hit the dirt with a crack. Everything was black, and I was still trying to process what had just happened. I knew from experience that a sound that loud—and that close to me—must have been a gunshot, but I wasn't sure whether I had actually been hit. I couldn't move my hands to feel around my head or neck. As my body lay limp on the ground, I couldn't feel any pain. I was numb and the adrenaline was still coursing through my veins.

The darkness that engulfed me seemed to be staying. I thought I was dead. This is it, I thought to myself. I had been gunned down and killed in a hole in the desert while washing my dirty skivvies. I guess I deserved it for not picking up my helmet or my Kevlar. It was the first time I'd gone into a gunfight with my head and chest completely open. I had never wanted to be one of those gung-ho Marines who had a complete disregard for their own safety. *A true hero's death*, I joked to myself.

Only I could laugh at the situation. Only I could see the funny side after almost getting myself killed running into open fire, or a poppy field, trying to draw out the Taliban. The cliché that your life flashes before your eyes seemed true at that moment. My mind conjured up images of Bobbie lightly tapping her stomach, telling me that our lives would be changed again by the little boy growing inside her. When we had found out we were having a boy just two hours before I headed out for the tour, I remembered her telling me that I had better make it back, because she didn't want to be a single mom. I could imagine her giving me so much shit for not putting my kit on, and not thinking about her.

I remembered the day the recruitment officer drew me into signing by doing pull-ups on the door frame of the office. I remembered the silence that fell over our dorm of young Marines in Camp Lejeune, as we watched the smoke billowing from the Twin Towers, and knowing that we would be going overseas far earlier than we could have ever imagined. I remembered the precious few weeks in between tours, where we would hop between bars, drink too many beers, and get thrown out on our asses. I thought of holding Bobbie in our backyard and watching the sunset.

Then I remembered being a kid, running around trailer parks in Ohio, stealing shit with my sister. I thought of all those books I had tried to read when I was too young, and all the trouble I would get into in school. What if I had decided to become a priest after all? I could have been preparing a mass, or reading the bible, from the safety of a church.

As I lay in the darkness on the dirt, four thousand miles away from home, I knew that if I wasn't dead, she would kill me for not putting on my protective gear. How stupid was I? As Forrest Gump would say, quoting his mother: "Stupid is as stupid does." I could have stopped for just a split second to grab my helmet. Did I have time? Would my friends be dead if I had hesitated and didn't distract the sniper? I guess I would never find out.

I was still blacked out a few seconds after I went down. I was in my own no man's land in my head. I felt like I was floating. I was directly under the sun in one of the hottest places on earth, and I weirdly felt cold and numb.

The Taliban did not have the skill and precision of our Marines, but they did hit their targets. Their weapons weren't as powerful as ours, but they could still inflict devastating damage on whoever was on the receiving end. Their snipers were better trained than the normal foot soldiers waving AK-47s above their heads while running around villages looking for Westerners to kill. A stationary target was right in their wheelhouse. A Marine was a great scalp for any terrorist. It would be something to brag about to all their fighter friends, and would be a badge of honor for their family, if they had any left.

Any luck I had managed to build up during my tours around the world, and during the many times I had been fired at, seemed to have run out at that moment. What had I done to deserve this? Is it because I abandoned my pregnant wife so I could fight for my country? I could never have imagined that I would die in the sweaty asshole of the world with a hole in my armorless body.

The few seconds I was knocked out seemed like hours had passed. I still had no idea what was happening to me and whether I was hurt. Suddenly I started to regain my hearing. First I heard my own breathing. It started slow, but it quickly gained pace. I started to hear *pop, pop, pop*. Then I realized I could open my eyes. I tried to peek at the outside world and squinted at the sun shining directly at my face, as if it was only a few feet away.

Marines around me were standing over me and firing back at the mud hut where the shot had come from. Dirt was flying everywhere and bullet cartridges were falling down by my side. They started hitting the floor like raindrops in slow motion, but then they sped up.

The other members of my platoon were standing over me, screaming to each other. They were barking orders that I couldn't quite make out. Then I could just about hear someone screaming: "Bee's down! Bee's been hit!"

I came around and opened my eyes a bit more, letting a sliver of light in. I slowly moved my hands over my body with any strength I had, and realized I couldn't feel any blood. If I had been shot, I would have been able to feel the dampness coming from the open wound.

I lifted my head slightly and realized I had already been strapped into a stretcher, and they were taking me to a helicopter to get me out of there. How long had I been out? I managed to see my torso and quickly realized something: the bullet hadn't hit me, but apparently it was pretty damn close. I looked up and saw the wall I had been standing against. On the top, there was a huge crater pretty much exactly where I had been standing. The sniper's shot had hit the bank only a few inches in front of me, and the blast of the dirt had propelled me backwards.

As I became more aware of my surroundings, I was suddenly engulfed in shadows. Lying flat, I was lifted off the ground to the sounds of "go, go, go." I felt like I was floating.

I fully woke up on a stretcher underneath a plume of green smoke. My squad had thrown down smoke grenades as they carried me out, in the middle of the gunfight. The battle was at its fullest intensity. The Marines were responding the only way they knew how, with full and unapologetic force. The medics and the other Marines evacuating me thought I was unconscious. They didn't know I was fine, just a little beaten up and a little shocked.

I tried to get up from the gurney so I could tell them I didn't need their help, but as soon as I tried, a huge arm came across my body and held me down. They weren't going to let me move an inch until I got to safety. Squashed down, I shouted at them, "What the hell are you guys doing? I'm fine."

I tried to jerk my head around to get their attention, but they were focused on getting me out as fast as possible and weren't giving me much notice.

One of the guys looked down and said: "Are you hit? Where have you been hit, buddy? You okay?" "

"I'm fine," I said again.

"Are you sure you're not hit? You got shot. I saw it.," a medic told me.

I shook my head, smiled, and said to him, "Almost."

He smiled back, but the Marines carrying me kept on running. The adrenaline was slowly returning, and I peeled my eyes open fully. I started to feel the heat again and the sweat returned. It was made worse by the group of fully grown men in combat gear huddled around me, jogging and sweating.

My fighting instincts gradually started to kick in as I regained consciousness. I was desperate to rejoin the fight, and my response to the flurry of bullets was to grab my gun. I reached down to my side, and it wasn't there. I had dropped it when I fell.

"I'm perfectly fine," I said. "I have a headache, but I'm fine. I need to get back out there." Someone next to me heard me and replied: "You crazy asshole. There is no fucking way we are letting you go back. You are out of here. We will take care of it from here. The guy who shot at you will be dead in a few minutes. We have them outnumbered. The chopper is on the way to get you."

"Dude, I'm not leaving my guys," I barked back at them.

So, they sat me up in the stretcher. They supported me by the shoulders, making sure I still had my balance, and then slowly lowered me down and sat me up against a wall. I was still breathing heavily and was still in shock. I was relieved that I was still alive. How the fuck was I still alive?

As I lay slumped against a wall, I stared up into the blaring sun. I still wanted to run back, grab a gun, and start shooting, but I knew I would get stopped or fall over from exhaustion before I reached the wall. I asked the doctor for some Tylenol and swallowed them without needing water; I didn't want to waste any time getting back out there. I needed to get back to work.

It was still chaotic. Marines were standing everywhere, firing back into the row of huts. I could hear the bullets flying overhead. A few hit the sand around me, but none were making the same dent as my shot. I could call it "the shot that almost killed me."

As I looked around, I noticed someone who wasn't a Marine. It looked like he was reloading his gun, but what he was holding was a lot smaller. Through my blurred vision I noticed it was a camera. It was Goran. I smiled at the fact that he was still playing with his equipment.

I saw him looking at the screen on his long lens, and he had a massive grin on his face, bigger than what I had seen before all hell had broken loose. He then caught my eye and started laughing uncontrollably. I was glad he thought my near-death experience was funny. He was a Serbian war photographer who had seen more conflict than most grunts, so his sense of humor had been slightly tainted over the years.

Still smiling, Goran walked toward me and started saying something. My hearing was still coming back to me, so I couldn't quite make out what he was talking about. In his broken English, I heard him say: "Bill, Bill. You okay man? That was fucking close man."

I told Goran I was a little shaken, but there were no cuts or bruises—nothing serious anyway. I barely had a scratch on me. It was a miracle, considering how close the bullet had been to my head. His concern didn't last long. Instead he turned his camera, so the lens was facing away from me and I was looking at the screen. "Fucking look at this," he said. I tried to focus and had to wipe more sweat from in front of my eyes. I finally made out that it was a picture of me. I was standing in front of the sandbank just seconds before the shot.

"I was testing my new lens. It takes a series of photos quickly. Look what I got," he said, still laughing to himself. I flicked through the images and was amazed at the shots he had taken. He had captured my brush with death in amazing detail. They showed me up against the wall, with my rifle primed, but my head and upper body exposed.

The first picture showed me getting ready to fire. The second showed the sandbank blowing up in front of me when the sniper's bullet hit. The third showed me turning my head away in shock, while shielding my eyes from the debris. The next two were me falling to the ground, with my gun still next to me. In the last image I was down and didn't look like I was getting back up. That's why the Marines thought I had been hit. That's why they thought I was dead.

Still a little shell-shocked, I told Goran the photos looked great, but I didn't really know what to think. I looked at them again. I could see the sand flying everywhere after the shot hit. I could see my arm covering my face in a flash, as I fell backwards from the pure force of the bullet. It was like a slow-motion action shot from a film. I tried to imagine myself as a superhero, dodging a bullet. But I was no superhero—I had just gotten lucky. Very lucky.

"I am a fucking Serbian," Goran said. 'I would never get pictures like that. These are ridiculous. I could win a Pulitzer Prize, but they would never give it to a Serbian." I still don't know if he ever got one. He told me he had seen photos like mine before, but of an American soldier in Korea. "How is that guy doing now?" I asked Goran. "He died," he said back to me.

Flicking through the photos on Goran's camera, I could see the funny side of what had happened. For some Marines, laughing was the only way to deal with the thought that you could die at any second. I started laughing so hard that tears started rolling down my cheeks next to the drops of sweat. Grunts were crouched down beside me, giving me the strangest looks. Eventually, we called in an air strike on the building and the firefight subsided, and I set what had happened aside, so I could carry on doing my job.

The next day our platoon got a call over the radio for me. The photos had caused quite a stir back home—they had been published in newspapers and even flashed up on the networks. They were perfect for the media campaign in the U.S. They were proof that the forces were showing no signs of letting up, despite the fact that the number of casualties were piling up.

Senior commanders called me in, and asked if it was okay for Marine public relations officials to release my name to the media, along with some details of what had happened. I agreed, reluctantly, but on one condition: I had to call my wife Bobbie and tell her what had happened, before they were published. I was already dreading that conversation. I knew exactly what she was going to say.

I was too late. I should have known that she had already seen the pictures. She was at home with her parents in Pennsylvania, when she caught a glimpse of them on an online forum for military families I had told her to follow. When I left for the tour, I had made her promise to avoid the news, because the TV coverage and articles made the situation look far worse than the reality. She was scrolling through the comments like I had advised her to do, and she clicked on a post that read: "Where was his helmet?" She immediately recognized me and started to scream uncontrollably, overcome with the terror that our unborn son would never get to meet his father. Usually, Bobbie could pretend I was training—as a coping mechanism—and never let herself think that I was in Afghanistan, but when she saw the images it suddenly became real. Her cries were so loud, her mom and dad ran up the stairs and found her pointing at the computer screen, and trying to speak when she couldn't. She almost went into early labor and collapsed into her dad's arms, knowing she wouldn't know any more information until I called her a few days later.

Everyone else in the world thought I looked like a hero, but her first question to me was: "Where the hell is your helmet and Kevlar?" She screamed so loud I held the phone away from my ear for a second.

She was mad, and rightly so, especially as she was carrying my unborn child. I hoped she didn't go into early labor as a result, but a few seconds later she scared me to death: she told me that when she saw the pictures, she felt a jolt unlike anything she had experienced, and didn't know whether it was the baby, or just a severe physical reaction to seeing me dodging a bullet. If she had given birth at the moment, she would have been madder at me for not being there. She switched between furiously telling me I was a dumbass, to saying how much she loved me and wanted me to come home.

"From now on, you wear your gear all the time. I don't care if you are doing your laundry, eating, or going to the bathroom. You wear your damn kit. Do you understand me?"

CHAPTER 10

On the night of May 18, 2008, just a few hours after my near miss, we sat laughing and bullshitting during our downtime in the compound. The shot was already in the back of my mind, and I was focused on the next task, whatever it was. We still had more work to be done, and my brush with death wasn't going to be a distraction for me or the squad.

As the evening went on, a sergeant I called Bump came over and told me he was going to check out the building where the shot came from. Our guys were going to stay on post, and Sergeant Peterson's squad were going to act as the react team in case anything happened.

When night fell, the guys started heading south, down the wall I had been standing against to the edge of the village, so they could then move east and push towards the sniper's compound. They weren't even three-quarters of the way when the rounds started coming in thick and fast. The first thing we could see was bonfires. The Taliban had started fires all over the area, knowing the flames would make our night vision goggles turn green, and our vision would be screwed.

I gave Lance Corpral Stanborough the call sign Sweetums—after the hairy ogre in the Muppets, who carries a club and has huge eyebrows and a low-hanging jaw—because he was a six-and-a-half-foot-tall monster. We gave him an M240 medium machine gun that were made to be fired from a tripod, that he could just carry around with a two-man team.

During the firefight, he did something I have never seen anyone else do: he picked up one of the thirty-pound machine guns, put it effortlessly on his shoulder, and cut the militant in half from forty yards. It was one of the most astonishing things I had seen in the Marines, but the shots kept coming, and I couldn't stand around watching in awe.

One of the squad leaders who was out there froze in panic and stopped moving forward. The sniper team noticed that the guys were pinned down and still being lit up, so their leader said: "Fuck it, we are going in to get these guys out." The squad leader then took out a frag grenade to throw into one of the Taliban bunkers we called Mouseholes (where the enemy would knock through a hole in a wall that was big enough to fit their gun muzzle so they could fire from a protected position). As he moved his arm and hurled the grenade into the air, one of his team leaders shouted: "Thumb clip, asshole!" On a grenade the pin isn't the only safety; there is also a thumb clip that holds the pin to the spoon. He had forgotten to take it off, meaning he had just thrown a completely inert grenade at the Taliban.

Ten seconds later, the enemy, hunkered down in the bunker and firing at us, were kind enough to throw it back to the squad leader, but this time the grenade was live. Luckily, their throw was off and it didn't hit anybody, otherwise it would have been a horrific mistake that cost us a man. But everything was still stalled; there was nowhere to go, and the sniper team knew they had to do something. They started heading north through a cornfield to try to flank around and open fire from another position. They started moving, and that's when scout sniper Lance Corporal William Justin Cooper got shot two hundred yards away. I saw him go down while there were five men stuck and still under fire outside the compound. I turned to Gunnery Sergeant Carlos "OJ" Orjuela, and started begging him to let my guys get out there to fight or go and help Cooper.

"I can do something. Please!" I asked him.

"No, somebody's got to hold down the building, and you're it," he hit back.

A few seconds later, we got a call on the radio from the outside that there was a casualty designated "urgent surgical," which means "without immediate medical attention, he's going to die." It was Cooper—he was hit bad, and time was already running out for him.

I turned to OJ again and said: "Look. I have my guys in reserve who can go out there and help. I'm going to grab him and bring him back. One of my fire teams can go out there."

"No, I can't let you go, but I can send Campbell." He ordered us to stay and cover the compound.

I turned and grabbed Campbell—my first team leader—and told him to go out there and get him back. They pulled out a poleless litter, which was essentially a piece of tarp with handles that can be used as a stretcher. It was a nightmare to carry someone, but the speed with which they ran out, grabbed Cooper, and brought him back while the Taliban were still shooting at them blew my mind. These guys didn't even blink. It was a moment that made me immensely proud, but I would have rather been out there with them.

They hauled ass back into the compound with Cooper in the tarp, and laid him on a platform that was a little over a foot off the ground and was used as a bed. The sniper team corpsman came in and started working on him, but he was in bad shape. He had been shot in the head, and the injuries were devastating. He was twenty-two years old, from Eupora, Mississippi, and had served two tours in Iraq before arriving in Garmsir. From what I heard, he was one of the best snipers in the battalion. I had nothing to do with my team at the time, so I decided to help the docs trying to save his life. I could hold the flashlight or just give them morale support; I didn't care, I just had to do something, anything.

He was the first man I had ever seen or known that had gotten hurt, aside from the Marine who was injured by a radio battery that exploded in a fire. I could still hear the firefight not even two hundred yards away, and the medics were doing everything they could in the pitch-black compound. I still felt like I needed to do something more to help. Then I saw his hand just hanging beside the platform. I grabbed it and put it in mine, and I just started talking to him.

Even though he was hit, I thought he still might be able to hear me, and some quiet words might be able to comfort him. Maybe he was still there and fighting for his life, like the men looking over him.

"Hey Coop, you'll be fine. You'll be fine. It's going to be okay," I kept saying, but his hand was stone cold. There was no movement; there was nothing. I knew he was still alive, but more life was being sucked out of him every second.

They tried to do a nasopharyngeal to get an airway through his nose, with a tube that goes down into the throat so he could breathe, but it didn't work. So the doc said he was going to have to perform a cricothyrotomy. He took a scalpel from his trauma bag, made an incision just above Cooper's Adam's apple to make a hole in his throat, and then inserted two hooks to open it up. The blood started welling up out of the hole. I was witnessing by far the worst thing I had seen in my life. I was still holding his hands and talking to him to try and calm him down, but he still wasn't reacting to any of the treatment. It was a dire sign.

The helicopters finally landed outside the compound, ready to get Cooper out of there. The two squads had pulled back from the bunkers in the firefight, and our guys took him out so they could try and take him to safety. The medics kept working on him, right until the last second when he was lifted up into the night sky. I stood and watched the birds, and prayed that by holding his hands in that dark place, thousands of miles away from home, I gave him some hope, some comfort, some fight to try and pull through.

It wasn't fifteen minutes later that we got one of the worst call signs a Marine could hear over the radio: Fallen Angel, for a Marine killed in combat, with his name William Cooper and his blood type. We heard "Fallen Angel, Fallen Angel" followed by his initials "WC" and the last four digits of his social security number. It was the early hours of May 19, 2008, just a few hours after I had almost been killed by the sniper shot. That was it for all of us—the level of rage was indescribable. The STA (Surveillance and Target Acquisition) sniper team was definitely messed up, and all we wanted to do was go back out there and deal with the Taliban members responsible for the first kill most of us had experienced. But we couldn't, because the last guys who had gone in and tried to push had been ambushed.

Instead, our air officer said he had ordered some Cobras, and they were heading our way for a strike on the bunkers and the surrounding buildings. We told them that whoever was in the building was responsible for killing of one of our snipers. Normally, the air strike would include a five-hundred-pound bomb and some smaller gunfire, but this time they were coming in with all the firepower they could. They were our payback. The first Cobra came in with hellfire missiles, and the second came in with mini guns, and for ten minutes they just battered the building with everything they had. After that, there was nothing but a smoldering ruin where those Taliban fighters had been. The most horrendous forty-eight hours in the Marines up to that point had finally come to an end.

The following morning we woke up still reeling from what had happened. It hit me harder than I could have imagined, but we still had to pick ourselves up and keep doing what we were there to accomplish. We were preparing to hit and clear another bazaar in Garmsir. They took our platoon up to the building that was the company COC at the time, and we staged there with another team who was going to roll through the other side of the bazaar. There the command police sergeant—who was responsible for getting you toilet paper and bringing ammo out to the range—had two fifty-five-gallon oil drums cut in half made into barbecue pits. He had bought a cow from the local butcher for about thirty dollars and cut it up, and was serving steaks to everyone who was coming in.

The next day we got word that we would be pushing into the bazaar that night. Our squad was walking through a graveyard when we noticed an Afghan man just sitting there on his own in the dark. He looked like he was asleep, but there was no way he wouldn't have woken up with seventy Marines approaching, even if they were being quiet. It was made even more scary by the fact that, at that point, we hadn't interacted with any locals; everyone we had seen was Taliban. We crept up to him and I told Campbell that we were going to search him, when he suddenly stirred and started screaming. He stood up and started trying to fight Campbell with his arms flying everywhere. Something just seemed really off with him and his attack techniques were not effective. He then tried to touch one of Campbell's knives, so Campbell jumped back. We all had our guns on him and we were ready to start firing, but I told everyone to stop shouting and calm the fuck down, so I could bring in our interpreter to try and make sense of what he was saying, or figure out what was wrong with him.

The translator tried to calm him down and talk to him, but even he was having problems communicating. In his broken English, the interpreter said: "He's not all in the head." I realized he meant the man was mentally handicapped. We had no reason to hurt him, and we also couldn't get any intelligence from him. So, we gave him some of our ready-to-eat meals and a pat on the back, and we left him in the graveyard so we could carry on. Within twenty-four hours, we found out from another patrol that the Taliban had found the mentally handicapped man and beheaded him, because they assumed he had helped us by providing information. It just added to my rage. These bastards had absolutely no mercy, and would even execute a helpless man in the most violent way possible, if there was even the slightest chance he had aided Americans. The man couldn't even speak, and the chances of him giving us reliable information was next to nothing.

We carried on, and set about clearing every building on the main street of the bazaar that was made up of nothing but mud huts and garages. Everything was locked, but we had to rip open every door and destroy every padlock, to make sure the Taliban wasn't hiding anything. They could have stashed weapons or IED materials anywhere. Our platoon hadn't moved ten feet when we heard a boom, caused by one of the Marines opening a garage door that had been booby trapped with propane tanks. The charge went off and he was flash burned. (He survived and was flown out, but ended up being medically retired in a burn unit in San Antonio, Texas.)

As we walked through the bazaar, the Marines would take the supplies left behind by the Afghans who fled, but we would pay for them: if we went into a building and found a carton of cigarettes, we would throw a twenty-dollar bill down and then lock the building back up again. We made sure the families who had fled would have a little something for their missing merchandise, if they returned.

It was relatively quiet, and nothing we found concerned us until Campbell suddenly told us to stop our patrol. He saw a deep freezer up ahead that was wrapped in chains with a lock holding them together. He immediately got a feeling that something wasn't right about it, which gave me goosebumps because he was an expert in explosives. We called in an EOD team.

They arrived straightaway—they had been expecting us to find explosive devices during our search, and had already put on their bomb suits so they would be ready to go and check it out. We held back as they slowly walked down the road to go and inspect it, making long strides in their heavy boots. They spent twenty minutes looking over the deep freezer, and they didn't like it either, so a member of the team attached enough C4 on the lock to break it during detonation. He walked away and blew it, barely doing any damage to the deep freezer, but enough to crack it open. I watched as he walked back, and was expecting a huge explosion when he opened the door, but when he looked inside he just started laughing and waved us forward. It was full of cans of grape soda, and we just started laughing at the fact we thought some pop might kill us. We picked up a couple of crates, dropped some dollar bills back into the freezer, and then carried on.

The operation was definitely a success. We found a building with some IED-making material that had not yet been fully rigged, and another with a cache of dozens of weapons, mortar rounds, and ammunition for RPGs. It had gone relatively without a hitch until we reached the last building, at the very end of the road. We breached the door, and one of the creepiest-looking men I had ever seen was standing inside. He had one eye clouded by cataracts and was unnerving to look at, but we ignored his appearance and went through the same routine of every facility we had cleared. Our platoon commander said we were going to take the building, we would give him one hundred dollars in return, and we would get him out of the area to safety. He would lose, but we needed the building, and to protect him from the Taliban.

Without flinching, he said, "No you're not. You're not taking my home." We told him that wasn't an option and it was going to happen anyway, but he was standing firm, and wasn't at all moved by our threats. We also needed the building because nothing else around had a good field of view of the rest of the bazaar. Rambo, our interpreter, said he would talk to him and make him take the money. Suddenly, we saw Rambo had the man up against the wall with a knife to his throat, telling him to take the payment and walk away.

"What are you doing," I shouted at him so he would release his grip. It seemed to work: the creepy man took the cash and left. As we searched the building, we realized why he was so determined to keep it: out back was a field that must have been ten acres of nothing but weed. Marijuana, along with opium and heroin, was a huge source of income for the Afghans and the Taliban, and there were mountains of it in Helmand Province. We had just kicked a man out of the home where he must have had millions of dollars' worth of weed, for a hundred bucks.

"Holy shit," I said to the guys, who were laughing at the ridiculous amount of drugs in front of them. Then I pulled them together and said: "Do not touch any of this or I will kill you—that goes for all of you." We'd worked with Afghan soldiers and police officers who were high in combat, and if my men took any, they would be in no shape to fight. After searching the rest of the building, we were sitting in the field, and one of the Marines started laughing so hard he was almost crying, and I thought he had disobeyed my orders.

He said to me: "Sergeant, come here and check this out." There was a herd of sheep walking through the field and eating every plant they could see, and after a while they started laying on the ground or jumping for no reason. They were high and had just decimated millions of dollars' worth of weed.

We stayed in the building for a couple of days, and after clearing it out, it was like somebody had flipped a switch. The three firefights we were getting into a day had ground to a halt, and locals kept flooding back into the area. We were no longer in constant battle mode and instead, interacted with the locals by handing them cash if their buildings had legitimate damage, and doing some census patrols. For two weeks we just dealt with normal people who had been forced from their homes. For us, the operation was a chance to bring down the level of psychosis and adrenaline that had built up, during the endless battles and the heartbreak of watching Cooper die. My near miss wasn't even a consideration, and I enjoyed just getting to know the locals in an environment where we weren't being constantly shot at.

We then got word that we were being pulled off the front for a break, and heading for Forward Operating Base Delhi in Garmsir, which was under British control at the time. We arrived in a seven-ton Armadillo covered in three-inch plating, to an unimpressive base that was about four thousand square feet and only had two small areas: one where the British Princess of Wales Royal Regiment slept, and another where the Royal Regiment of Scotland slept, and they wouldn't talk to each other. They had a forty-two-inch TV turned to a music video channel that just played the Ting Tings' song "That's Not My Name" over and over again, and a few board games, and that was it. We had no idea what good five days in this place was going to do for us.

We were bedded down with the Scots, and the first time working with them was a linguistic adventure. I couldn't understand most of what they were saying, but when they started drinking, it was a whole different ball game. It just reminded me of Robin Williams' sketch on drunk Scotsmen from his stand-up routines.

Then we were sent out to The Rock—officially called Operation Post Rock—long considered one of the most haunted places in Helmand Province. It was a thirty-foot-high mound of dirt overlooking poppy fields and the Amir Agha villages, where you could hear unexplained voices, strange lights at night, and random waves of radio static. It also constantly smelled of rotting corpses. As a military position, it was a perfect outpost where we could see the Taliban, but underneath the surface of the mud were tunnels that led to a tomb, or so we were told. The locals had buried their dead in the mound for years, and they believed it was cursed. We carried on going from building to building for census patrols: asking people what their names were, what they did for a living, and where they were from.

I received orders from my platoon commander to prepare the squad for a mission at 2 a.m. one morning, during our stay at The Rock. We went to bed about 6 p.m. the evening before to squeeze in a couple of hours of rest, but at 10 p.m. there was an enormous explosion that woke me up. The smaller blasts were no longer enough to even stir me in the night, after countless gunfights. The radios roared to life with Marines asking if they knew the situation, or where the point of origin was. Nobody knew, so after a few minutes of an adrenaline spike and preparing for action, we just went back to sleep and prepared for our patrol just a few hours later.

On patrol, we went past The Rock and were halfway through one of the villages, when we came across a hole in the ground that was at least eight feet deep and twenty feet wide. We called in the EOD team to do a blast crater analysis, to find out what had caused the hole, but a few hours later, one of the dogs—that followed us around and became our so-called mascots—started walking over to us.

"Um, what's the dog got in its mouth," Campbell asked me, pointing at the scraggly mutt. I couldn't tell what it was at first, but as he got closer, I noticed what looked like fingers hanging from his teeth. He was chewing on a human hand.

"What the hell, where did you get that?" I shouted at the dog and took it from his mouth. The hand had been completely shredded at the wrist and there was nothing else. *Of course this is happening at The Rock*, I thought to myself as I stared at the hand in disbelief, not knowing what to do with it. While I was considering whether to just drop it on the floor or take it back to command, the dog started heading back towards the crater, and I knew if we followed, we would find something else. It ran over to the edge of the hole and started chewing on a ribcage with nothing but just the bones. I kicked it off and I started getting even more of a creepy feeling, before the dog charged off to another patch of dirt where there was just a puddle on the ground with a man's fake Rolex lying in the middle. It took me a second to realize that the puddle was his melted skin suit, with the bones completely dissolved. We didn't know if he was with the Taliban, or just helping them. Then, for some deranged reason, I just started laughing. Maybe the deployments had finally gotten to me, and the death we encountered every day had just become part of my conscience, or maybe it was the fact that the knock-off watch he had probably bought for less than twenty dollars was still ticking. Campbell was waving his hands trying to get me to shut up, and pointed to the twenty village elders standing on a hill about twenty feet behind me, just staring silently. There were also banknotes scattered around what was left of him. I laughed harder.

The EOD found that the fake Rolex man had prepared around five hundred pounds of an ammonium nitrate and aluminum powder mix, a deadly mix of fertilizer similar to what Timothy McVeigh had used to blow up the Alfred P. Murrah Federal Building in Oklahoma City in 1995, killing 168 people. It would have cracked a tank in half if he had used it effectively, but it blew far earlier than he anticipated. He had put the charge in the ground and connected it to the power source before he attached the trigger made of BBs and Styrofoam. The explosion would be initiated by two of the BBs connecting, and he didn't realize two of them were already touching. The bomb blew while it was in his arms and the blast was so powerful it blew the bones out of his skin. The investigators picked up the skin that made up his face and tried to plump out the features, so it could be run through facial recognition software. None of the locals recognized him even though his face was intact. We never worked out if he was working for the Taliban or on his own.

It was my first experience with an IED and the horrific damage it inflicts. Luckily it wasn't to any of our men. It would be a couple of years before I would learn first-hand what damage the horrendous explosives left by the Taliban could inflict on me. But it was only a couple of days before I would learn that the people I had grown up with in the Marines, who were still fighting in Helmand, were far from safe.

CHAPTER 11

On June 26th, 2008, Bobby told me over the phone that Staff Sergeant Christopher Strickland had been killed by a roadside bomb in Helmand, while working as an EOD technician. We had gone through the school of infantry together, graduated in the same class, and were in Camp Lejeune at the same time, though he was in third platoon whereas I was in second. It was the first time I had ever hung up the phone on my wife, as I really couldn't deal with the news. His son Mike was three years old at the time, and his wife Carrie was good friends with Bobbie. It hit me even harder when we found out our tour of Garmsir would be extended by a few months after July 4, to show some of the British Marines around before we left. I managed to raise a smile when I asked one of the Brits how it felt to be barbequing T-bone steaks with Americans on Independence Day, and he turned to me, laughed and said, "Shut the fuck up, man."

After we found out we were staying in Afghanistan, Ethan was born. It broke my heart, knowing I could have been there if I had been sent back earlier with the advance party as anticipated, though I wasn't the only one who had a kid at that time. But I found out the news in the most amazing way: Bobby sent a printout of photos of the little man, and our battalion commander got a convoy to travel ten miles through Indian country—with the mail and a phone—to hand-deliver them to me. I would spend the last few quiet weeks, waiting until the day I would get back to Bobby and meet my son for the first time. There were no firefights and little contact to be worried about—we were just going through the motions until we got on the flight to Shannon, Ireland, and then homebound for the U.S.

On October 18, 2008, I finally landed, and there were no words to describe seeing the woman I had been thinking about constantly for eight months, and my little man for the first time. They met me at the airport with Charlotte and Kelly, two of my best friends from high school, and she drove me home and walked me in the front door to a sign covered in Ethan's painted footprints that read: "Welcome home, Sergeant Bee. This is the first time I get to meet Daddy."

Though I was happy to be home, I started self-medicating with alcohol to deal with everything that had happened in Garmsir. Cooper still weighed on my mind. When we got back to the U.S., we would sit through what we called "don't kill yourself" classes—hours of PowerPoint slides that taught you how to recognize PTSD in yourself and the Marines around you. I knew I was going to have issues after the deployment, especially with the firefights, the close call with the sniper, speaking to Cooper as he slipped away, and after hearing Strickland had been killed. I was hypervigilant, I was sensitive to loud noises, and I would have random adrenaline spikes. It was the start of a long journey.

The Marines, after more than two hundred years, were starting to recognize and treat mental health problems in their ranks—they told us if we had any issue, that it was okay to talk about it. Looking back, the classes helped me in ways I hadn't ever imagined they would, as what had happened in Garmsir had put a heavy load on me. I was sent back to Twentynine Palms in California again, to train for the next deployment, when I first ran into what was called the red room. It was a simulation of an IED blast where paid actors, including those with multiple amputations, would recreate the aftermath, and medics would have to go in with the Marines to treat them. It was so intense—seeing all the bodies lying on the floor and the noises and the smells—that I tapped out after about forty-five seconds and told my platoon commander I couldn't do it anymore. I then went out to Coronado for the Joint Fires Observer training course, where I would be able to call in and coordinate air support from AC-130 gunships and hardcore artillery. On my first night in our quarters—at about

1:00 a.m., when I was in that perfect state right before falling asleep—everything around me suddenly exploded, and the sound of machine gun fire started filling my room. I jumped straight up and ran outside, thinking artillery shells were coming for the base in San Diego, of all places. However, I found they were just doing live fire obstacle training by my window. It was my first flashback, and it scared the shit out of me.

We started our workup for the next deployment in December 2009, when President Obama told the West Point cadets in his commencement speech that 30,000 additional troops would be sent to Afghanistan. There was going to be a major surge in Helmand Province, including on the Taliban stronghold of Marjah. There had been talk of going to Iraq, which excited me because I'd never been. But I was still pretty pumped when we found out we would be in the next wave of troops heading back over Christmas to take on the Taliban. None of us wanted to spend a tour in Japan, sitting on a boat in the middle of the Pacific, or training other countries how to do our job. We wanted to be where the action was, and all the guys wanted to do was pull their triggers. I knew it was going to be a hard fight and I was ecstatic. The problems I had faced after returning from Garmsir didn't really crossed my mind.

My squad was more prepared than any of my other tours. There were fifteen men who had been through the most realistic combat training in the Marines, and they were hungry to get out there and get the job done. They were a mix of new guys, grunts who had been with me in Garmsir, and senior team leaders who were all bloodthirsty, and I trusted them. As I was getting ready in my living room, Ethan—who was about one-and-a-half years old at the time—was going through my gear, handing me my equipment and helping me put it in my pack.

While we were waiting for the bus—after Bobby had already left—I was joking with the wives of one of the other Marines, and trying to scare the crap out of her. I told her that all I wanted for Christmas was a new set of legs, knowing the Taliban had started using IEDs more frequently against Western forces. Our squad took a flight heading east on a double-decker civilian aircraft, and managed to sneak into first class, while the battalion commanders and company commanding officer went up the stairs into business class. A poor young lieutenant came down to try and kick us out while we were being treated like kings, and we told him to get lost. For twenty-four hours, we sat in seats that could recline into beds and had their own TVs, while the rest of our guys sat in coach class.

After a short stay in Kyrgyzstan again and a stopover at Kandahar, we went on to Camp Bastion, the main base for British raids and operations in Helmand Province. It was being developed into a huge complex for thousands more troops. We then went back down to Camp Dwyer where we would start our staging. First, though, we went up to Fiddler's

Green, a farm ten miles north of Marjah where the newer Marines could get some combat experience: get shot at a couple of times so they would know what it felt like, before the real fighting began.

Right off the bat, the fighting was far more intense than in Garmsir, and the locals didn't want anything to do with the Marines. It was a shady area, and I already had a bad feeling that the opening part of our tour wasn't going to go so smoothly. After a few days, we were moved to a building around seven hundred meters west of us. Our first mission was with the first platoon squad, to the north of a dried-out irrigation canal—or wadi—just outside our new compound. We had gotten intelligence that the Taliban had stacked the area with IEDs, because they knew we'd used them for cover when the bullets started flying. We were back to clearing buildings again, and were the react team giving cover to the Marines ahead of us. As soon as we started moving, we received contact from another building to the north. It wasn't much, and sounded like it was just a couple of guys who had spotted us and started shooting. I took my squad to the north side of the building, to where the gunfire was coming from, and we opened up our magazines and the response stopped. They must have seen our firepower, and decided they wanted to get away and head back north, but we couldn't chase them because I was still covering the first platoon squad, which was getting bogged down by heavy contact from all sides.

My men then stormed the building, but most of the Taliban who were inside had already gone. We knew they had been inside for a while, because all we found inside were heroin, poppy seeds, marijuana, and any other narcotics you could think of that they could use as currency. All that were left were two older men, who my squad started questioning to find out where the fighters were going. I left my men to try and extract more information, and started walking around to see if they had left anything else behind. I poked my head out of one of the doorways and saw four men standing in the middle of the sand, with a rocket-propelled grenade launcher sitting between them. I was stunned, because the Taliban were experts in hiding and you would rarely see them. It was a tactic they used to their advantage, from when the British first invaded in 1839 to when the Soviets arrived in the 1970s. They would build a little mouse hole—big enough to stick their barrels through—shoot a few rounds, and then run to a different position. During firefights you could only see muzzle flashes, never their beards, their clothes, or their facial expressions.

They were only around three hundred yards away. I got excited and thought to myself, *This is amazing*. I felt like a little kid at the candy store. I knew I could have easily dropped each one of them with my rifle, but something possessed me and I shouted for the AT4—an eighty-four-millimeter anti-tank rocket that you could throw away once it had been fired.

I had only used one of them five times in my career up to that point; they had all been on the range, and it had only worked one time. They would often be a dud, and there were loads of safety features to go through, including pulling out a pin in the back of the rocket, that most forgot to remove.

I was handed the AT4, and I cradled it for a second as I watched the four men just standing around, as if nothing was going on. They had no idea I had them locked in. I yelled "rocket" to warn everyone around me I was ready to pull the trigger. I took a deep breath and pushed my finger down. Nothing happened.

"Goddamnit," I shouted, and went to grab another before I looked down at the rocket. The transport safety pin was still in. I had made the same dumb mistake so many Marines had made before me, but it was still ready to be fired, so I steadied myself again, yelled "rocket" for the second time, pulled out the pin and fired.

It was a one-in-a-million shot that landed dead center in the middle of the Taliban men and sent them cartwheeling through the air. I was possessed again and I started laughing. I spiked the rocket on the ground like a football and then held two middle fingers up at them, before the rest of the guys yelled at me to get back to cover, because we were still being shot at. I later found out from one of our interpreters that the man I killed was a local Taliban commander, and it made the shot that little bit sweeter. While the rounds were cracking around us, our platoon got out of the building and tried heading north along a thigh-high wall, but we were pinned down, and we realized we couldn't advance any further. The shots were coming from all sides. I was sitting alongside my friend Lieutenant Malone, when a tracer bullet hit six inches down the wall between him and me. When the round dropped to the floor it was still burning green, and he turned to look at me with the widest eyes I had ever seen. I had just escaped another close call, but I just started laughing again and told him, "They can get a hell of a lot closer than that."

We were pinned down, so I called air support to tell them we couldn't maneuver and we couldn't withdraw. The firefight had been going on for a relentless three hours at this point, it was dusk, and the men were drained from keeping up the fight, even though they couldn't push forward. Two Cobras flew in and performed a "show of force" by dropping flares. It was anticlimactic, but did a good job of scaring the Taliban away.

We hiked back to the building we were staging from, and we were so tired from the firefights that we didn't hear the sound of the Taliban firing anti-aircraft guns towards our patrol. All we could hear was a weird buzzing noise that sounded like a hyped-up bumble bee, and I thought nothing of it. Luckily, they were a thousand yards away and had no chance of hitting us with a piece of equipment they weren't used to. When we got back, I played it cool by telling the guys to take their time and relax. For many of them, it was their first firefight, and I told them their adrenaline would be insane to the point that, when it came down, they would start shaking and they would freak out. I reassured them that this was perfectly normal and there was no reason to be scared. In the calmest voice I could, I warned them that they were going to see a lot more firefights, and they would have to deal with the physical and mental reaction every day. I left them to recover and walked into the squad leader's room, where I felt something I had never experienced before. As soon as I sat down, I started shaking. I had never been through it in Garmsir, where we were fighting at three hundred yards away. This time we were shooting at men just fifty yards from us. The combat was closer and more intense than I could have predicted. These Taliban weren't running either. Normally, as soon as we laid down the firepower they would flee, but this time they were staying put, and kept fighting until we brought in air power.

It was only Day One, and I remember turning to the other men and saying, "None of us are going to leave this place alive. This is different."

On day two, my squad was sent out to help snipers Ben Parker and Rob Richards set up in what was called a hide in a building, to keep watch over Taliban movements near our compound. Their job wasn't just to shoot bad guys, but be hidden and call in airstrikes without being compromised.

That's why they were called "Scout Target and Acquisition." We were back to knocking down doors to check if anyone was inside. My squad was working in tandem with another: we would enter one building, give it the all-clear, and they would move up and hit the next one. It was going smoothly until we hit the second or third building, when our guys started to push east out of a building, and had only moved ten yards when a man with an AK-47 opened up on us, from right in front of our position. Aside from the compounds around us, it was just open fields and no cover, so finding a position to return fire from was a harder task. I knew he was in another building just across from us, but we couldn't tell where he was inside, so we got behind a wall and unleashed hell back. However, we still needed to find a position for the STA team. So when the Taliban's firing trailed off for a second, we moved to a second location, closer to the building we needed to take. Now, all there was between us and the target was a 150-yard field, with nothing to hide behind. It was going to get ugly. We were being closely watched by the Taliban, and I knew this open stretch of land was terrible to try and run through, but we had no other option. It was our only path.

I got the team leaders together and told them to just blanket the area in smoke grenades, while we hauled ass across the field to try and get to the other side. I got ready with the rest of the men, and one of the Combat Cameramen with our team looked at us in a way that said, "What the fuck are you doing?" We had a hundred pounds of gear on us, we were in full Kevlar, it was 120 degrees, and we were going to be running faster than we ever had in our lives.

We just took off into the abyss, and for the first fifty yards it was smooth. Then the Taliban brought in the heavy fire, and we could see the rounds cracking off the dirt by our feet while we were sprinting. It gave me the biggest adrenaline boost of my life, but we couldn't slow down. All we had to do was make it to the other side. With our heads down and our packs rattling behind us, we made it to the compound and dove inside, somehow with none of us getting hit. We turned around to give cover fire for the rest of the men, so they could move up, and I decided to clear the building where the gunfire was coming from, with grenades. It was the first time I had ever thrown a frag in combat. All of us tossed them, and blew a hole in a door that had been covered with bricks, to try and stop us getting in at all costs. We barreled through to the east side of the empty compound, and I could see the building we were targeting for the STA team. The only thing in between was another fifty-yard run in the open fields that wasn't going to be any more fun than the first sprint. So my team put our heads down again and ran for our lives, and dove into the next doorway to find an old, spindly Afghan man sitting there watching us. He could have been anywhere between age forty and ninety, because those locals did not age well in the heat and the impoverished conditions, and he must have been left behind when the younger soldiers got away. Inside we found four hundred pounds of ANFO (a mixture of ammonium nitrate and fuel, the illegal but perfect cocktail to make a powerful explosive). The old man didn't say much to us as we placed him in flex cuffs and took him into custody.

With the squads still under heavy fire and cut off from any escape, we called in air support from an F-18 to send the Taliban scurrying back to their holes, and we managed to get back to our main compound, after another intense day of gun battles. Then, we had what we thought was a reprieve. Charlie Company came to replace us in our position so we could go down to Camp Dwyer, but less than forty-eight hours after they arrived there was a fatality—the first in our battalion in the trip, and another sign that it was only going to get far worse. The Marine stepped on an IED pressure plate when he burst through a door, and the explosives hidden in the walls killed him where he was standing. Since dealing with Cooper's death in Garmsir, I hadn't faced much more death on the battlefield, and it was hard for everyone. For three weeks we sat at Dwyer and trained a platoon of the Afghan National Army, to try and get them ready to take control of the area, so we could leave. They were natural fighters whose ancestors had been surviving for two thousand years in the face of invading forces with more modern technology and advanced warfare— but when it came to professional military training, they were the worst to handle. They were corrupted like the government they were fighting for, all spoke different languages because of the varying tribes they were from, and there was no morale. We tried to teach them the correct military ethos and how to use our weapons and equipment, while the senior officers were stealing from the junior soldiers.

The only time they ever showed unity was when they cooked together, or got into dance-offs with some of the idiot Marines. One of them was Lance Corporal Kielin Dunn—a small, nineteen-year-old Marine who would get on the floor and start spinning on his head, with a huge smile on his face that made everyone around him happy. He was an incredible break dancer, and the nights where we were all together— relaxing, laughing, and telling jokes—were among my best memories of what was a horrendous tour. We were away from the action for a little bit and got to act like we were having a wild night at a bar at home, without so much drinking. Those were the brief moments of joy, before what would be the fierc- est and most heated hit of my career.

The squad leaders gathered for a company brief that was more intimidating than anything I had been through. This was nothing like the worst-case scenarios we were warned of in Garmsir. We were handed detailed photos of the Taliban defenses, including trench systems, where anti-aircraft guns were located, and positions where they were suspected to have portable air defense systems—the top end of their arsenal. This mission would be as real as it gets in Helmand Province, and when I told the squad what they could expect from the next mission, they knew it was scary. Unlike Garmsir—where we had to stuff bullets into our pockets and tape them to our pants—we had all the ammunition and the grenades we wanted. I was handed a radio specifically used to call in air support, and a laser that could be seen for one hundred nautical miles, that could communicate with bombers and help them zone in on their targets. The high-tech equipment didn't do a lot to help boost our confidence, because we knew they were giving it to us for a reason: we were going to need it.

We were ready to go, and were told that night that D-Day would be in less than twenty-four hours. The next day came and went, and nothing happened. Another day passed, and once again, our trip was cancelled at the last minute. Our battalion was just waiting to get the go-ahead, and it was always postponed. We were constantly on standby until early February 2010, when Gunnery Sergeant. Brian Walgren addressed The Marines of Alpha company and fired us up with a speech that has gone down in Marine folklore. It was based on a debate in 1974, between retired pilot and former astronaut John Glenn and Howard Metzenbaum, his opponent in a race for Senator of Ohio. Metzenbaum told Glenn he wasn't qualified to run for Congress because he had "never had to meet payroll." Glenn responded with an attack that left his rival speechless. Walgren repeated that attack, and added a few details relevant to the adversary we were about to face. Walgren quoted from Glenn's speech:

> I served twenty-three years in the United States Marine Corps. I fought through two wars. I flew 149 missions. My plane was hit by anti-aircraft fire on twelve different occasions. I was in the space program. It wasn't my job; it was my life that was on the line. And this wasn't a nine-to-five job where I could take the time off to take the daily cash receipts to the bank.

Walgren repeated Glenn's request to Metzenbaum to have him visit a veterans hospital to see "the men with mangled bodies" and "look them in the eye and tell them that they never had a job". Walgren then quoted more of Glenn's speech:

> You come with me [to the hospital] and visit any Gold Star Mother. You look her in the eye and tell her that her son never held a job. You come with me to the space program and visit the widows and the orphans of Ed White, Gus Grissom, and Roger Chaffee [the astronauts who died during testing for the Apollo 1 mission in 1967] and you look those kids in the eye and tell them that their dads never held a job. You come with me on this Memorial Day weekend to Arlington National Cemetery, where I've got more friends than I would like to remember, and you stand there and you watch those waving flags and you think

about this nation and you tell me that those people never held a job.

I'll tell you, Howard Metzenbaum, you should be on your knees every day of your life, thanking God, that there are some men who have held a job and they required a dedication of purpose, a love of country, and dedication of duty that was more important than life itself. Their self-sacrifice is what made this country [fucking] possible.

Walgren added his own words: "You all know damned well—you all get out there and you fucking do shit. Because of the Marine to your left and the Marine to your fucking right. God, country, and Corps don't matter at that point."

He finished by saying: "You're going to do what you need to do for fucking each other. Not for anybody else. And [the mission is] tomorrow...you can't fucking stop us now. What the fuck are they going to do now?" We were pumped up and prepared for what needed to be done. We had been stood up so many times waiting to be shipped out, but this was it.

CHAPTER 12

D-Day for the assault on Marjah was also the day before Valentine's Day, 2010. My squad was part of the first wave of helicopters was and tasked with setting up a blocking position to the east of a bazaar. I got my guys into the back of the V-22 Osprey and followed them in last, so I could be the first one off when we touched down. The target landing zone was a large poppy field that we were told was good and dry. As we flew, I looked out of the windows and saw tracer fire aimed at the other aircraft with Bravo company—flying in formation within us, but heading to a different landing zone. It sent chills down my spine, because if they were shooting at them, they were more than likely aiming at us, and we had no control over our fate in a helicopter. We were like sardines in a can, stuck with no way to escape.

I jumped off the back of the helicopter, and when I landed, I sunk into thick mud up to my knees. It was the worst landing zone I had ever seen, and I thought, *Shit, this is going to be bad,* but I still had to shout to make sure my guys all got off. One by one, they got off, and I watched as the lower halves of their bodies disappeared beneath the surface of the muddy field, and they started to wade through it with their 150-pound packs on their backs. It was horrendous, but there was nothing we could do; we had to get to the bazaar before the second wave of helicopters came in. The Marine carrying the machine gun ammo for the squad leaped off the back and landed awkwardly. He was almost bent in half with his momentum taking him forward and the weight of the pack dragging him back, and he fell to the ground and started screaming in agony. They quickly got him back on the Osprey to fly him out, and I later found out he had broken his back.

Our battalion air officer—Captain Smith—came over, grabbed me by the shoulder and said, "Bee, we've got to get the guys the fuck out of this landing zone before the rest of the birds land."

"No shit, sir," I said back. "But my guys are all down and we can't move." We managed to get out of the way by the time the second wave landed, and then the third. The company got together and by the time the sun came up around an hour later, we were aware of how much of a disaster the arrival had been. One of the men in the second squad came up to me and Sergeant Cage complaining that there was something wrong with his knee, and he cut away his cammies and showed us it had swollen to the size of his head. He'd ripped his kneecap so he was also out—we'd already lost two men within the first two hours of the mission. As it started to get bright, we set our sights on the bazaar, which was a ghost town. It was silent, and our first kill was a dog that startled us when it ran out of one of the houses, heading toward us. We made our command post a building that looked down a row of shops split by a dirt road and a ten-yard-wide canal, and then another row of shops, that we had to clear before we could set up our blocking position. The first seventy-two hours in Marjah were filled with violence, with a few Marines shot and at least one killed. The offensive was already starting to make headlines, and the U.S. was ready to show that we could put a new government in place with the Taliban emptied out. But we knew the reality was that this was going to be more vicious than anything else encountered during the war.

We hadn't even emptied two buildings on our first patrol when the first rounds of gunfire started cracking around us from just one hundred yards, and it was so close it even intimidated me. I crouched down behind an oil drum, which admittedly wasn't the best cover I could find, as the squad hit back in anger with their own hail of bullets. During the chaos Gunny Walgren came over and tapped me on the shoulder and—as if nothing was going on—said, "What are you doing down there, Bee?"

"What are you doing standing there?" I said. "This place isn't a joke. This isn't like our last firefights, these guys can shoot."

He was carrying a cup of coffee and didn't seem fazed by what was happening. He said, "Ah, I'm good." As soon as he said it, a round passed about two inches above his head. It was so close I could feel the wind from the bullet, and he dropped straight away. Then I spotted the two-story mud building they were firing from, surrounded by two-and-half foot walls that were missile-proof. But one of the men in my squad fired a round straight in the middle and it collapsed, sending four Taliban men running into the open in a daze.

"Light 'em up!" I told the machine gunners. They dropped them with four hundred rounds of ammo and the firing stopped. We got them. We found a building in the bazaar to take a breather and assess our position, and I told my guys that no one was allowed to get past us, no matter what. The Taliban were sending local farmers to try and push through Marine lines, and figure out where they could position IEDs or send in explosives in vehicles, including one man we shot and killed when he refused to listen to our demands and instead put two middle fingers up at us. One of our STA sniper teams found the only four-story building in the center of the bazaar with the best view of the surrounding area, and settled in for the day. They rarely miss—every five minutes we would hear a single shot we knew was another insurgent who wasn't getting to us. I think they got twenty kills that day and the rest of us didn't have much to worry about.

For the next two days in that building, the only encounters we had were the Taliban just taking long shots at us, trying to figure out our positions. Nothing came close, and we were able to go back to the command post for a few days to act as a react team. Most of the guys were grateful to be back in the base for a few days, because every time we left there would be endless gunfights. We were helping stack the thousands of water bottles and food packs that helicopters were dropping at night, because trucks couldn't deliver supplies, for safety reasons. The bottles would explode or scatter everywhere when they hit the ground, and—because they arrived at night—the water would be hot when you went to drink it the next day. The work was bullshit, but for some a welcome alternative to being under constant Taliban fire. However, any sense of calm could be shattered in just a few seconds.

It was February 18, and we got a call for a casualty who needed to be evacuated from the third platoon's position, where I had been just a few days before. I immediately got scared. It was the break dancer, Kielin Dunn. He was just a teenager and he had been shot in the head. I got a few of my guys together in the back of an MRAP vehicle, so we could go and get him and bring him back. We ran behind the truck. As we reached the bazaar, we found Dunn on a roof with blood soaking the bandage around his wound, and I could already tell he was slipping away. The Marine with him called in the casevac, got Dunn off the roof, got back up, and got behind a machine gun and unleashed hell back at the Taliban. He kept firing back towards the building while he waited for our help to arrive. He took a round in his Kevlar vest, but the plate stopped it, so he kept firing while rounds were coming at him from all sides. He didn't get down until the Taliban shot and hit his machine gun.

Memories of Cooper came flooding back to me as we put bandages over Dunn's eyes, put him on a stretcher in the back of the truck, and took him back to the command post. In the truck, I held his hand and started talking to him like I did with Cooper. I told him everything would be okay, but from the looks of his injuries I knew it would not, and he wasn't reacting to anything. They went to do a cricothyrotomy, or "cric", on his neck, but the doctor hit the wrong spot and went through his voice box, and he started to aspirate. A second doctor came in and tried again, and did it flawlessly, to try and get the air moving again. The helicopter arrived to pick him up, and I just hoped by some miracle they could get him treatment in time at Camp Dwyer. Just a few minutes later, we got the Fallen Angel call again.

His death floored me because he was so young, and he was the sweetest kid. I read later that he told his mom that he wasn't afraid of dying and that if he did, it would be with honor. He told her—on calls and on Facebook—that it was rough in Marjah, but he had to stay strong for the rest of us, and he was. All of us loved him and we were all impacted. The situation was not fine—a kid who was just eleven years old on

9/11, and was now not even old enough to go into a bar with us, was lost—but we had to carry on.

Night fell just a few hours later, and the Taliban hit again from the building from where they had shot Dunn, in what was only my second firefight in the dark, after my first deployment in Kandahar in 2002. We had picked fights when the sun went down in Garmsir, but this was different, as they were bringing the heat to us. I told my commanding officer that we needed to deal with the bad guys inside, and would do it with my first order to cause death and destruction from the air. I found out there was a flight of A-10 Warthogs nearby, loaded with rounds big enough to decimate a tank, so the mud building wouldn't stand a chance. I briefed one of the pilots and we watched as they swooped in and opened up their guns, and the structure exploded. There was then a group of secondary explosions, which meant the Taliban must have been storing something lethal inside. I never found out how many guys were inside, but I knew there were many and that they were no longer a threat.

After Dunn's death, the push across Marjah continued, and—as a show of force—the higher-ups got all of the companies to march across the desert on a giant line, for a photo op. Tactically it was ridiculous, because the Taliban could have laid down a series of IEDs in front of us, but the Marines wanted to show the world the insurgents had been cleared from Marjah, which wasn't entirely true. It served no purpose for us, and we knew the reality of the situation in this part of Helmand Province.

That's why—in April 2010—we took up our final position, which became home for the rest of the deployment. The temperature was becoming unbearable again during the Taliban's springtime offensive, when they came in with ferocity to harvest the poppies and pay off all the local farmers, who looked after their drugs during the winter. Our squad seemed to be getting in more firefights than any other, and every patrol was a gamble. There were a couple of areas around our compound that were very dangerous, including a gas station we called the Taliban Biker Bar, that always had sketchy men hanging around. It was surrounded by canals, so it was hard to approach without being spotted, and every time we were caught, the men would come out and drive away on their mopeds and bikes.

We were getting intelligence from informants all the time: locals who would tell us how many guns the Taliban had, what type they were using, and how many there were of them in a certain place. Some of the locals liked us, but others only respected us if we broke down their doors and raided their homes. There were local rivalries between their neighborhoods and between the two main tribes—the Pashtun and Dari—which made patrols in the area complicated, but we knew the militants were still there and had their eyes on multiple Marine scalps. I spent every day one week turning over a local man's mud house, because we believed he was running guns, but he was as clean as a Mafia don. We couldn't find any weapons every time we searched, and he got so angry with us tearing down the carpets from his walls, and putting holes in his thatched roof, that he left. The evidence suggested he was innocent, but I always thought he was hiding something. I was angry and—after Dunn—I stopped caring about the mission. All I wanted to do was get the guys out of the area and safely home. I didn't want to lose anyone else.

To the east of the Taliban Biker Bar was another gas station, where we would get into a firefight every time we went on patrol, and afterwards the men inside would flee. I decided to set up a small raid from an abandoned building beside it. A group of around fifteen men set off at 2 a.m., and my boys made it inside without making a sound. They were like ghosts, even though they had one hundred pounds of gear on their backs. We all packed into a room that couldn't have been much bigger than the living area of a trailer, and made sure they stayed silent while I went to check the rest of the compound, where we found the components for making an IED. I knew right away something bad was going down. At 9 a.m., we poured out of the building and prepared to blitz the gas station, so we could scare the hell out of the men inside.

One of the engineers cut a wire holding the door closed and we burst in, shoving our guns in the locals' faces and shouting at them to get on the ground. They had no idea what was going on. Some of them tried to run and hop on their motorcycles, but we didn't let them get away. We put a couple of the men in flex handcuffs and found one of them had ten thousand dollars in cash. We broke some of the locks of the doors inside, but found nothing. All of a sudden, we started taking rounds from every direction. It was an ambush.

The Taliban had snuck a machine gun to a canal—just fifty yards in front of the gas station—in the middle of the night, and were attacking us from all sides. We were struggling to fight them off. The men we had detained ran out of the back of the building when we turned to start firing. Our machine gunners to the north and west were trying to fight them back, and we were firing rockets at them. There were explosions, shrapnel was whipping past us in every direction, and fifty-gallon fuel cans were starting to leak. It was insane. We managed to take cover behind a knee-high wall outside the gas station, and then I thought to myself—for the first time in my career—that I was no-shit going to die. A piece of shrapnel hit me, but luckily it was just a cut.

I called in a mobile reaction team from the combat outpost to back us up, and when they arrived Lieutenant Malone screamed, "Indirect fire." Our Marines were shooting at us because they couldn't see us. The private running point had assumed our muzzle flashes were the Taliban, so they opened fire in our direction. The squad that came to back us up had Mk 19 grenade launchers, and one of them landed eight feet away from me. When the fighting subsided, and the private who I knew was responsible rolled up in a truck, I dragged him out and wanted to kill him. He was just excited to get out from the base and into the action, so he opened up at the first thing he saw. But there is no excuse to open up on your own men, because if you aren't sure who you are firing at, you don't pull the trigger.

We went back to the canal where the Taliban had put the machine gun and found drag marks, which were probably from the bodies of the men we had gunned down. They would always take their dead away quickly because of Muslim burial rules, and because they didn't want us getting our hands on any remains. We started following the tracks, heading towards a building not one hundred yards north of us, when rounds started coming at us yet again. A bullet tore through the calf of a corporal in front of me, and we all dropped to the floor. It was the first time someone in my squad had been shot during one of my deployments, and I was furious. The rest of the guys started to return cover fire, while I got on the radio to call in a helicopter to get him out of there. He was bleeding everywhere.

Pedro, the pilot coming in, could land on a dime. He didn't care what was happening on the ground when he came in, but I wanted to give him some cover with smoke grenades. I took out the first set and threw them straight into a muddy field, so the purple smoke just splattered into the water. I tried a second time, while mimicking Nicholas Cage from the film *The Rock*, where he holds his arms outstretched with flares in either hand, and signals for incoming helicopters on Alcatraz. I sparked the smoke grenade cans above my head, ran over to the landing zone, and guided Pedro in to take the injured Marine out, while my hands started to burn.

We turned our attention back to the building, and planned to attack it from the side by making a hole with one of our rockets. Winston landed a round right next to an AK-47 laying on top of the wall and caused it to disappear, but he made a perfect entryway for us in the thick mud that we rarely were able to penetrate. I told the guys to throw a frag inside to clear it. One of them threw first and a few seconds later, when it blew, I heard women and children start screaming, and my heart sank. I had no problem hurting or killing Taliban, especially because of the way they treated people, but I never wanted innocent bystanders to be collateral. I told the rest of my men to try and put the pins back in, but we couldn't. My heart sank even further and I started thinking that I was going to end up at the military prison at Fort Leavenworth. I told the guys to throw them because we were almost out of options. We still had to clear the compound and we would be the ones blown to pieces if we kept them in our hands. The screaming continued as the rest of the frags exploded one by one, and then my squad and I burst in to see what was inside. The first room in the compound was empty. But we knew there was at least one Taliban in the area, so we searched the rest of the room and found the screaming women and children had taken cover in a back room, too far away from where the grenades could do them any damage. They were all fine, but it scared the hell out of us. We went up to them while they were cowering and huddled next to each other, and tried our best to calm them down with the help of our interpreter. A few seconds later one of my men told me he found two military-aged males hiding in another room of the compound, and they looked like they could be Taliban. It was like a switch flipped inside me. I went from caring about the mothers and the daughters we could have killed, to rage and to focusing on getting back at whoever shot my friend.

I got our interpreter, stormed into the room the two men were in, took out my pistol, and put them on their knees. I was livid and had lost any sympathy I had for these men.

"Look, I know one of you shot my boy," I screamed at them. "Which one of you is going to talk, and which one of you is going to go missing?" The interpreter joined in and started telling them I was crazy, and I would kill them if they didn't answer. What neither of them knew was there wasn't even a round in the chamber, and I was just trying to scare the information out of them. Then—as I was shouting—one of them looked at me and smirked, and I snapped. I punched him in the face as hard as I could with my thick Oakley Kevlar gloves, and he dropped to the floor. The impact was so hard I broke a bone in my hand and got what is known as a boxer's fracture. We dragged the two men out of the compound, and Lieutenant Malone saw the face of the man I had just smacked.

"Holy shit Bee, did he get hit in the face with some frag from a grenade?" he asked me.

"Yep, that's how it happened," I said without hesitation.

It was 6 p.m., getting dark, and we were all exhausted from a day of constant gunfights. We had to cover just four hundred yards across open fields to get to our compound for the night, and we hadn't even run a hundred yards when the shooting started again. I fell to the ground and felt the pain surge through my hand when I landed. We'd had enough for the day, so we walked back to the compound in a peel formation, where three of the men returned fire while the fourth moved backwards towards our final destination. We made it back and I took off my glove and saw that my hand had swollen up to the size of a balloon. The only issue it gave me for the next few days was that it was hard to go to the bathroom: that was the hand I used to hold the plastic bag I would pee in.

Meanwhile, the intensity of the fighting didn't subside, and it didn't look like we would be heading home any time soon. We would run across open poppy fields while rounds flew overhead, getting just a few hours of sleep before the sun would come up, and it would start all over again. It consumed all of us and it was unforgiving, but we still had a job to do in this shitstorm of an operation. My focus was still on getting my men out alive, and I was thinking more about getting home. I would call Bobbie when I could and check in on the moments in Ethan's life that I was missing, but sometimes my family life would be forced onto the back burner by the ferocity of the battles and the complete focus they demanded.

There were also points in Marjah where I felt like my Marine career was turning into *Groundhog Day*. My hatred for the Taliban and their culture only intensified when a local father came up to us, claiming we had killed his five-year-old daughter and shot two of his cows. He came to one of our command posts and said, "Do you know how much those cows cost me," and didn't mention his little girl. To them, girls were a possession and an investment for the future, when they could be sold to older men as their wives. It reminded me of a moment in Garmsir in 2008, when I saw a girl—who couldn't have been much older than nine—covered in jewels and wearing a dress, getting ready to marry a fifty-year-old man. The interpreter told me she would be a mother by the time she was thirteen. In those moments, it was hard for me not to take my gun out and shoot these men on the spot, because they filled me with so much fury. It set my attitude for the rest of the time in Marjah. If the Afghans didn't care about their own, I was only focused on my Marines. We saw the worst of humanity every day. Wives would try to give us information just to get away from their abusive husbands, and some of the

Marines would see men beating women with broomsticks or anything they could find.

We were in the same village as the sketchy Taliban Biker Bar, on the northside of one of the irrigation canals. Our squad was spread out moving forward, when we suddenly heard shouting coming from the buildings on the other side of a set of walls that were only fifteen yards away. It seemed like the Taliban was going through the village and clearing it out themselves—it wasn't a good sign. I got on the radio and told my squad to stand firm and take cover where they could. I found a spot behind a wall right next to what looked and smelled like a sewage trench and got ready to open up, when the machine gun fire came in thick and fast.

I poked my head out to look east towards the gas station when I saw a fighter with a blue head scarf lying on the ground behind a Soviet PK machine gun. I was staring right at him and could see the expression on his face and almost the glint in his eye. He was so close. I was ready to fire back at him when he pulled the trigger, and suddenly 2008, the sniper, the round inches from me, and the sandbank bursting all flooded back to me. It had happened again; the only difference was I was behind a vertical wall this time, not on top of a horizontal wall. The bullet from the machine gun smacked into the mud right next to my head and I dropped. The sound was the same and the round was as close as it had been in 2008—I just didn't have a photographer crouched beside me when it happened. I had escaped another brush with death, and gotten lucky yet again. I took a few moments to compose myself when Matt jumped on top of me and started screaming.

"Holy shit, Bee, are you okay? Are you okay?" I could see the panic in his face as he desperately tried to figure out where the round had got me. I started laughing and he looked at me like I was crazy. I was, but I was fine.

"Holy shit, I thought they smoked you in the head," he said back, while I was still chuckling underneath him. "That's twice now!"

"Tell me about it," I said, as the machine gun rounds kept flying past our heads. We tried to figure out the best way to get away without being exposed to the incoming fire. I got up and composed myself while the wall beside me was still taking a beating. I saw the sewage trench beside us. I looked at Matt and we both knew that was the only way to escape. We jumped in and the shit reached up to our nipples. We waded through by holding the rifles above our heads, and the rest of the squad started cackling while the firing was still going on. When I got back to the compound, I decided against taking one of the normal Marine showers with a water bottle hanging from a rail, and jumped straight into one of the irrigation canals and started trying to get myself clean.

In March 2010, we set up a roadblock in an area where we knew the Taliban were running weapons, and were looking after an intersection that they ran with the Afghan police. We were merciless when it came to letting anyone through, and it was chaotic having to deal with the locals. The offensive in Marjah was supposed to have been led by the Afghans, and was named Operation Moshtarak—or togetherness—in an attempt to show that the locals were the driving force. Once the Marines had steamrolled the Taliban out of the area, the Pentagon planned for representatives from the Afghan government to come in and take control, but working alongside the natives was a constant struggle, showing how far they would have to go before they could restore order and maintain some sort of democracy in their own country.

When our squads would go in to replace the Afghan National Police, sometimes they would start shooting at us with a powerful fifty-caliber DShK Heavy Machine Gun, and they were meant to be on our side. Most of the local officers were corrupt, and we could never figure out why they were trying to disrupt us. Sometimes we were forced to fire back, but it was a miracle none of us ever got hit. They also made our lives harder by not doing their jobs properly or slacking off. Some of them would start fires that would blur our night vision, making it almost impossible to patrol and rotate with them at night. They also wouldn't pay attention to check the area around them thoroughly.

That all came to a head one night when we went to relieve a scout sniper team from the intersection. We took over from them and not even fifteen minutes after they had left us and were walking back, an IED went off. If the Afghan police had been paying attention, there was no way an explosive could have been planted there. The explosion ripped through the area. We ran towards the blast site, and when we got there I found Marine scout sniper Rob Richards had catastrophic injuries. Shrapnel was lodged in his legs, back, and left arm, and a huge nut the size of a quarter had flown into his throat. He didn't look good, and all I could think was that I was losing another Marine I knew. He underwent an emergency tracheotomy on the battlefield, and his foot was almost severed. A helicopter came to pick him up, and I felt reassured when a couple of hours passed and we hadn't gotten a Fallen Angel radio call. He'd survived by the skin of his teeth and was already looking at a horrific road to recovery. Richards was one of the best and bravest Marines I knew, but his reputation was ruined when in 2012 a video surfaced of his team appearing to urinate on a corpse of a Taliban fighter. He was court-martialed and demoted in rank for this incident, though it was found to be tainted by "undue command influence" (when the higher-ups influence the outcome of the proceedings). He should be known as one of the most skilled and deadliest scout snipers the Marines had at their disposal.

For us, the hits would keep on coming. The Taliban wasn't giving up and Marjah would be the last place on earth many of these Marines would see.

CHAPTER 13

In May 2010—as two of the other squad leaders and I got ready for another hit in Marjah—our platoon sergeant Staff Sergeant Hafner walked into the room of our combat operations center and said in a very matter-of-fact manner, "This afternoon, Sergeant Joshua Desforges of Bravo Company was shot in the head and killed by a Taliban machine gun." He was just twenty-three years old.

The staff sergeant turned and walked out, and my heart broke. Marine Joshua Desforges was a close friend; he hung out with Bobbie and I when we were at home in Jacksonville. He was a ladies' man and one of the funniest guys I knew. He went on a JFO training course with me and lived with two of the squad leaders—Madden and Rouser—who I'd spent hours with on deployment. I absolutely loved Joshua as a friend and a Marine. It hit Bobbie especially hard because she had gotten close to him. It was yet another reminder more men would be lost before we left Afghanistan. Madden escaped when a round ricocheted off his Kevlar while he was out on patrol, but we were getting reports of more men dying every day. We'd lost so many men, not just through deaths but through injuries. It was starting to wear everyone down, even more than the non-stop violence and constant exhaustion, which never seemed to go away. We were sick of getting into firefights, and we had reached the point where everyone was jaded and ready to go home. I started to go internal. I barely spoke to Marines who'd become my closest friends. I stopped cracking jokes. I focused on getting back to my family.

I was on patrol base when I got a call from Rouser, saying someone wanted to say hi to me at the base. We headed back and I found Derek Shanfield, a twenty-two-year-old Marine who had been recruited through my station while I was working with his older brother Sydney. He also had an identical twin brother named Devin, and at first I couldn't tell which one I was talking to. When I realized it was Derek, I was stunned he had already been made sergeant, less than five years after he'd signed up. He was with Zach Walters, another young Marine who had deployed to Afghanistan earlier than the rest of his squad, because they didn't have the same combat experience we did. They wanted their leaders to get some action under their belt—get to know the area that was extremely kinetic and seeing action constantly. Their squad had been deployed in the Mediterranean where they got a lot of training done, but it was nothing like a stint in Helmand Province, so we had to show them the ropes.

Their arrival was a sign that our deployment was ending, and all we had to do was make sure we survived a handful of patrols, before we could get back to the safety of a base and get ready for our flight back to the U.S. We had Shanfield or Walters with us every time we left the base, but I tried to keep them away from areas where we knew the Taliban would start a fight. I wanted to keep them close to our combat operations home. There was also a rule that the two of them were not allowed on the same patrol, as we didn't want their squad losing both leaders before their tour had even begun. We didn't want to take any risks, while we made sure they got accustomed to the surrounding neighborhoods and got to see some of the scarier areas we had encountered.

Our patrols for a couple of days came and went without any problems, and everything seemed to be fitting into place for a smooth transition over to the next squad. Then came June 8, 2010. During a pre-patrol briefing, both Shanfield and Walters volunteered to go on patrol to a small, sleepy part of a village where we hadn't seen any movement overnight. I agreed that they could come along, but reiterated to them again that we were not there to start a fight and that I was only showing them around. I explained to them that it was a building we had been to before, just south of the Taliban Biker Bar that was surrounded by ten-foot-high walls, that meant we could go in without being seen. Murder holes were also cut in, so we could see what was going on outside and fire through if needed.

The compound was similar to where we had been ambushed. I didn't want to send everyone in at once, just to be safe. We set up a satellite patrol, where one of the fire teams sat in overwatch while the others moved around. I walked in behind Gonzales, who had a metal detector in his backpack. I thought that I should really sweep the building and check for any devices potentially hidden under the dirt, but decided against it. We were only going in to take a look around, and I wanted to keep moving to decrease the chances of the Taliban sneaking up on us.

Our patrol team spread out inside the building, and I took Shanfield and Walters to a corner where you could see out towards the gas station—where we would always get attacked—and I started to describe what would happen.

"Every time you patrol this area, without fail you will start seeing mopeds and vans roll up." A few seconds later—as described—a cavalry of vehicles showed up, and I saw one of the men get out with a pair of binoculars and a radio. I knew he could have been a local Taliban boss, so I called over our marksman with a suppression rifle and got him to take him out. He went down, and then the marksman called me over to say his rifle had failed to chamber the next round. It infuriated me because it was a simple fix for anyone who knew what they were doing: he hadn't put enough lube in the barrel to pull the round out.

"What the fuck man? This is basic maintenance," I told him, and then all I can remember next was a hollow "thump" sound so loud I could feel it through every inch of my body. I was lifted off my feet and flew through the air until I landed hard on the mud floor. I was back in darkness. It had happened again in my career that had come to resemble *Groundhog Day*, with the same situations happening repeatedly. The world turned into paper straw, and all the Marines around me had become so small it was like I was looking through the roll of a paper towel. I didn't know what had happened and I tried desperately to regain my focus. The next few moments were a blur, and I can only recall a few flashes of Corporal J. J. Ponce saying: "Smoke the motherfucker on the moped." He had been in the building to the north of us and I couldn't recall when he had arrived. I had no idea how much time had passed, and everything that followed came in spurts of consciousness. I was in a helicopter being checked over by a man in a helmet. I couldn't hear anything and there was a searing pain in my head. Then I was on a stretcher back at base, running across what I think was a field. I woke up for a few seconds and freaked out, because I was trapped in what seemed to be a metal trash can, which I now know was an MRI machine. They dragged me out, and my memory started again, but my head was still all over the place. What had happened? Why was I only remembering a few seconds at a time? Why was I back at the base and why was I getting medical treatment? I still had no idea and didn't know how much time had passed.

At the moment of the explosion, 8,835 miles away, Bobbie told her sister she suddenly had a feeling something was wrong. She was in Pennsylvania for her nephew's high school graduation and her dad's birthday. At first, she blamed it on being nervous for the eight-hour drive back to North Carolina with two-year-old Ethan. She couldn't have been more wrong.

Finally, I woke up in a tent of the hospital wing of Camp Dwyer with two-thirds of my squad scattered in beds around me. Every time I opened my eyes I could see my guys bandaged up, including the one whose jammed rifle I fixed. He was being treated for horrific burns. His face was swollen and every few hours nurses would wheel him out for surgery so they could take more pieces of the building out of his neck. When I looked at the men around me hidden underneath bandages, all I could think was that it should have been me.

I sent them into that building; I was responsible for them. I should have had Gonzalez sweep for explosives with his metal detector and I should have made sure they were away from danger. All I could do was lie in that hospital bed with my whole body in pain, consider what had happened, and feel the guilt I would have for the rest of my life. I still didn't know the full extent of the damage and assumed the injured were just those lying around me.

I still couldn't figure why I was hurting when I woke up on the second day, in the hospital wing. I knew I had been caught up in some sort of explosion, but couldn't figure out why it felt like my brain was banging off the sides of my skull. I struggled to remember where I was. My memory of that hollow sound was still extremely spotty, and I couldn't connect the dots every time I tried to remember what happened.

A Navy Captain doctor, who told us he'd first served in Vietnam and was in charge of medical treatment in the area, asked us if there was anything he could do for us. We laughed and I said, "Doc. Every time we ask if we can go for a smoke, we are told no." He raised a smile back and he understood what we were going through, so he ignored his medical training and experience and said, "I'll see what I can do."

I would pass out so often. I couldn't separate dreams from reality, which is why I was stunned when I woke up in a hospital bed, and found a pack of Marlboro Red cigarettes on the small table beside me. A National Guard nurse said we could light them up in a small area with a smoke pit they'd set aside for us outside the tent, so we all wandered out in nothing but our scrubs.

Considering the circumstances, we were all very relaxed and were joking around as we enjoyed our cigarettes. We were laughing at the fact that just eighteen hours earlier we had been sleeping in dirt and eating Marine food packs, and now we had real lights, air conditioning, better meals, and women—but we were in a hospital, and I still didn't fully remember why. I turned to the only guys who could stand and had joined me for a cigarette, to try and find out more.

"God, I'm just sore all over today, and I don't know why," I told one of them.

He turned to me and said, "Are you serious? You really don't know? We got hit by an IED yesterday." That was the first time I fully grasped the catastrophe and figured out why we'd been taken out of the combat zone.

The Taliban had embedded two explosive devices in the wall of the building. Both of them had gone off and ripped through the building, and the body of the Marine whose rifle had jammed protected me from the blast when I crouched down to fix it, which explained the extent of his burns. I was more concerned about the guys that were still out there.

The second day of our stay at the hospital was when I started getting more information about the blast, and the men still out there, and reached the lowest point of my life. Our squad was hit by another IED a day later and one of the Marines had to have both his legs amputated. Now he was in the hospital beside us. The news I then received would change my life forever and send me into a spiral from which I would never recover: I was told that Shanfield and Walters were both killed by the IEDs that wounded me, and it was my fault. No matter what anyone else told me, I knew I was to blame. The blast was so powerful it decimated their bodies. All the remains of them they could find could fit into trash bags. Walters was just twenty-two years old and recently engaged, and Shanfield's family was very close to me. I had been tasked by their loved ones with looking after both of them. The wave of culpability hit me harder than the blast: I was the reason they were in that building, I was the one who decided to take them both on the patrol, and I was the one who decided against telling Gonzalez to do a sweep with his metal detector and ultimately find the explosive that killed them. All of the scenarios kept flooding through my head and repeating themselves. *What could I have done differently? Why didn't I hold one of them back at base? Why didn't I take an extra few minutes to check out the building?*

I lay in the hospital bed and refused to talk to anyone. Even the nurses struggled to get a response from me when they made simple requests. The battalion commanders would walk in and ask what happened, but what could you say when two Marines had been killed under your watch and it was your fault? A Lieutenant Colonel—who I wasn't a fan of—tried to strike up a conversation and I stonewalled him. He understood, but said something to me that I had never heard in the Marines up to that point, and it stuck with me: "You're going to need help because of this. You're going to need to talk to someone to get through this, and you don't need to be scared when you do."

Bobbie was on her dreaded drive home from Pennsylvania, talking to the wives of one of my Marines about how they were excited for our return in a month—on July 4—when she was interrupted by a text from another spouse that read, "There's been an accident." She hung up, pulled over, and frantically tried to get hold of the woman who had messaged, when she got an incoming call from Afghanistan—from me.

She picked up the phone, and I started to scream from both the pain and because I couldn't hear what she was saying. She could barely make out what I was howling when I cried out: "I'm coming home baby!" I tried to explain what had happened in a couple of words, but they were jumbled by the head injury and my muddled recollection of what had happened. A member of the medical staff stood beside me, and tried to calm me down as the emotions poured out uncontrollably. When we hung up, the Marine headquarters contacted me to confirm our address in Jacksonville, because they didn't think I would survive.

Still struggling to come to terms with what I had done, and knowing that this culpability would follow me for the rest of my life, I decided to write a letter to Ponce—while he was still on the front line—that essentially read: "Fuck the mission. I don't care what you have to do, but make sure the rest of the guys are safe. We have already lost too many men."

After four days of anguish in the tented hospital wing, shutting myself off from everyone around me, I learned I was being transferred to the U.S. military base in Landstuhl, Germany, so my brain injuries could be assessed. The blast had blown holes in my eardrums, and I could only walk a few yards before I lost my balance and toppled over, but the main concern was my head. My memory was still clouded in fog, and it seemed like time hadn't passed while I was in the tent. They call it shell shock for a reason: I would get flashes of minute details every so often, but then I would quickly get disoriented and confused.

My only recollection of landing at Bagram on June 13, 2010, was lying on a stretcher on the way to yet another medical tent, and looking up and thinking it was dumb to be surrounded by mountains that provided perfect firing positions for the Taliban. The base had grown to a military monster since the last time I was there in 2003, but what stuck with me was how we were fish in a barrel with two hundred foot hilltops around us. They took me into a plywood building and told me to stay inside until my flight out, but I was bewildered because they split me up from the rest of my squad. I was deemed "walking wounded," as compared to the rest of the guys, who were more seriously injured.

One day—during my short stay at Bagram—I needed some fresh air and went outside our hut for a cigarette, when we were hit by a rocket from a Taliban who had crouched on top of one of the surrounding hills. All hell broke loose, the air raid sirens started sounding, and everyone around me ran like crazy to one of the concrete shelters dotted around the base, that looked like pill boxes. While everyone was freaking out, I stayed put on the steps outside the building and happily puffed away on my cigarette. The rockets were one hundred yards away at the very least and I knew I was safe, but everyone else kept running to take cover. I didn't have any money for cigarettes, and I started to notice people dropping their packs as they ran, so I walked around and stuck them in my pocket while the rockets kept coming. I returned to my seat and popped another smoke in my mouth, when a man came sprinting over to me, dragged me towards the pill boxes, and tried to figure out what the hell I was doing.

"Are you okay, man?" he asked me.

"I'm great," I said back, with a crazy grin. "I got four cigarettes out of that. It's a great deal and I have no idea why the fuck you guys were running."

I was so used to those attacks that if it had happened on the front lines, we would have slept through it. Maybe I was going crazy, or maybe I was devoid of any emotions and just didn't care. Nothing fazed me by that point—all I could think about was Shanfield and Walters, and how I was responsible for what happened. I didn't know how many days passed at Bagram before I was on a C-17 to Germany, on one of the hundreds of stretchers bolted to the floor and lined up in rows, from the nose to the tail of the plane. It was a flying hospital with nurses and medical staff as the air stewards, tending to patients instead of passengers. I grabbed one of the doctors as he was walking past and asked him if I could have something that could put me to sleep, so he slipped me an Ambien. I was lights out until we hit the tarmac at the Landstuhl Regional Medical Center, where my new, abnormal life was about to start.

CHAPTER 14

I walked off the flight—with the help of medical staff—and into a tiny mountain village full of homes with red-shingle roofs, overlooked by the sixteenth-century Nanstein Castle. I could barely hear and was struggling to keep my balance. While we were being processed into the veterans' hospital, I got pissed off almost immediately, when we were asked to sign a waiver promising to refrain from alcohol. I had just left a Muslim country where drinking was illegal and non-existent, and I had arrived in the world's beer-drinking capital, where I was banned from having a pint at the end of the day. It was going to be tough for me to get through this without booze, having already used it as a form of self-medication. It was an escape that I too heavily relied on, but there wasn't much else to pass the time in this tiny community. To make things worse, when Bobbie called the base to find out if I'd arrived safely, she was told they had no record of me. She told me about it a few months later and it took years to get resolved.

They'd lost a full-grown Marine, and all my paperwork, in a screw-up that would cause even more problems in what was left of my career and my life, when I left.

I was confused by the donated clothes and blankets available for us to choose from. Why did the hospital have these creature comforts, when the grunts were on the front lines pulling the trigger, sleeping in dirt, and wearing cammies for weeks? I had left my guys behind to keep the fight against the Taliban going, and all I wanted to do was send them something warm. The doctors on base put up the service members with brain injuries—like me—in an officer's hotel where each room had a computer and a phone. It freaked me out, because less than a week before I had been fighting to get a sip of cold water and a meal that wasn't a ration. I had a string of appointments with specialists on my schedule, to take me through tests to find out the extent of my brain injuries.

Before I set off on my seemingly endless path of treatment, I went to find the other guys I knew from Afghanistan who had also been sent to Landstuhl—Rob Richards and Luke McDermott. Richards had barely survived the IED attack that left shrapnel in his neck. McDermott got a cricothyrotomy and couldn't talk, so he was communicating everything with a white board and a pen. I crouched by his bed and he wrote, "Where am I?" followed by, "Has anyone told my parents?" It was excruciating watching him suffer, and I tried to do everything I could to help him, until a Marine liaison came down and told me to let him do his job and handle it for them. They were trying to keep me focused on my appointments instead of worrying about my friends, despite the pain they were going through and the responsibility I felt.

During one of the first vestibular tests to examine my blown eardrum and find out why my balance was so bad, the doctors pulled out an inch of wall that had been wedged inside my ear canal since the explosion. That explained why I couldn't hear. The doctors then put me through a lot of basic exams to figure out the damage to my cognitive functions, and to fix the fact that I could still only walk a few feet before I lost my balance. They would give me a list of words I couldn't remember. The puzzles were meant for a child, and every time I walked away in fury because I couldn't complete them. Deep down I knew the solution, but my head wouldn't let me do it. I had no idea why. It got to the point where a nurse had to escort me to the appointments, because I kept getting lost and would end up in the middle of this huge hospital, disoriented and confused. The red flags kept coming, and I realized very quickly that something was very wrong with me.

But the most terrifying moment came when I was sitting at my computer, and suddenly the screen went black and I was thrust back two weeks into the building in Marjah. I was there, and it felt like it was happening all over again. I could smell and feel the heat of the explosion, I could see the Marines scrambling around me, and I tried to get up and search for

Shanfield and Walters. I felt like I was being dragged through the dirt to the stretcher. Then I snapped, and I was back in the hotel room, staring at the computer screen. It fucked me up. I felt broken, and it kept happening. I had lost control of my brain: every so often I was back in that building, smelling the heat and looking for Shanfield and Walters. It would stop me in my tracks, no matter what I was doing, and I could do nothing to stop it. I could have more say in the outcome in a gunfight with the Taliban, than with these attacks. It happened persistently for two weeks. The whole time I think I was in Germany, although I can't be sure exactly how long I was there for. I had lost all sense of time, and I struggled to piece together the hours of the day, let alone a week.

My stay had gotten so long, they considered flying Bobbie and Ethan out to visit, but I was desperate to get home. I had grown a mustache, and my traditional high-and-tight haircut had turned long and grungy. I begged the staff on base to get me to a barber, so I could at least look like a Marine, to try and feel some sense of normalcy. I bought $400-Oakley sunglasses with the money we were given for food and clothes, and had some real local beer smuggled in to me. I could enjoy it while the soccer World Cup was being hosted in Germany at the time. I wasn't allowed to leave base to watch the games in a pub with the European fans, but the atmosphere generated by the soccer fans around me, and watching the games on base, lifted my spirits. Meanwhile, the doctors were still trying to decipher what was going on inside my head that caused the vivid flashbacks. I knew whatever it was would follow me for the rest of my life, just like the deaths of Walters and Shanfield would. They were the demons I was going to face every day, while trying to decide the next step in my career with the Marines. Even though my brain was messed up, I still wanted to be punishing the Taliban with my squad for all the evil I had witnessed in Afghanistan.

It was a surreal day when I got the green light to fly back to the U.S., because my volatile psychological condition had still not been fully diagnosed. I was worried about how I would react when I saw Ethan and Bobbie. My son was barely walking when I had left for the Marjah deployment, and it was bizarre to think that he had been growing up while I was sitting in a mud hut or in the middle of a poppy field, six thousand miles away. After a flight into Bangor, Maine, a night at another hospital, and phone calls from Bobbie frantically trying to find out when I was landing, we finally arrived in Camp Lejeune. There was no way I was going to spend another minute in a bed on a ward. They called Bobbie to come and pick me up, and I was so stunned when I first saw her that I stayed in the car, until a Marine told me: "Dude, are you going to say hi to your wife and son?" I wasn't sure if it was my brain acting up again, the shock of being reunited with them, or the seemingly endless doctor's appointments already on my schedule. Ethan was shy, and it took a while for him to recognize the father he hadn't seen in six months, but when he and Bobbie hugged me, I was washed over with relief and happiness, even if it was only for a fleeting moment.

I considered joining the Wounded Warriors battalion for Marines injured in battle, but found I was surrounded there by men who needed far more help, so I went back to the 1st Battalion, 6th Marines. I wanted to deal with the doctors and the problems with my head on my own time, while still serving locally with the guys who were back home. Many others were still spread around the world. McDermott and Richards were still in Landstuhl recovering from their catastrophic wounds, and I tried to get hold of those who were still in Afghanistan or back in the U.S. I also kept thinking about the men who didn't make it back because of me. I was moved to limited duty when I returned to work, and was only allowed to do administrative work in a weapons platoon. All the while I was in rehab with more testing on my vestibular system, and still enduring flashbacks where I was back in the IED room in Marjah. The doctors would make me shake my head for ten minutes in different directions, and try to get me to balance on an inflatable ball to see how I reacted, and if I could keep balance. I would run one hundred yards during physical therapy, and either violently throw up or just fall over. I persisted, even though I had no idea if any of the treatments or medications were working, because I was determined to find out what was wrong with me. I was also taking MACE (Military

Acute Concussion Evaluation) exams, to try and determine whether I was experiencing concussion or traumatic brain injury symptoms. I said "yes" when asked if I had headaches, dizziness, memory problems, balance problems, nausea or vomiting, difficulty concentrating, irritability, and ringing in the ears. I would suddenly forget where I was while standing in the middle of the room, and get angry at the smallest thing.

I was thinking of Shanfield and Walters, and my decision that got them killed, at least once every fifteen minutes. In every flashback I could see Gonzalez's backpack with the metal detector in front, and I remembered deciding against sweeping the building because we wouldn't be there long enough. Then I'd see the men lying around me covered in burns and bandages in Camp Dwyer after the blast, and the whiteboard McDermott was using to try and communicate in Germany, after his leg was amputated. The brain fog meant there were days where I couldn't tell up from down, and I felt like an idiot. Hiding the rollercoaster of emotions and anger, so I wouldn't lash out at friends or family, made my recovery worse. The thoughts carried on all day, every day, and it gradually wore me down to the point where I turned to drinking again to self-medicate, and Bobbie reached her breaking point. She tried to get me help, but every time she tried to tell my Marine command I was having problems, they warned her that complaining could jeopardize my career.

It was September 2010, nine years since that day in New York that sparked the War on Terror, and accelerated my journey to Afghanistan to destroy the terrorists responsible. My fight against the Taliban had fueled my desire to go into every gunfight without fear, and to make sure I wiped the insurgents out of Garmsir and Marjah. Marines were still fighting and dying in Helmand Province, despite promises from the Pentagon brass it would soon be over, while I was at home battling a brain condition I still didn't understand. I knew I had multiple traumatic brain injuries, but that was it. I still hadn't gone through a full neuropsychological examination to find out the finer details of what was wrong with me, and my frustration grew every day. I still hadn't fully come to terms with the fact I wouldn't be able to serve overseas again, and the anger and dejection made me more alienated than ever. My depression, and constant need to get drunk to try and escape my dark reality, weighed down on my marriage.

The Marines I hung out with were dealing with similar issues, and we found ourselves racking up enormous bar tabs during insane benders, and breaking down with each other to talk about what was going on. For my thirtieth birthday, we rented a party bus fully stocked with alcohol—with a stripper pole in the middle—for a group of these friends to go from Jacksonville to Wilmington, North Carolina. On our way home, the driver pulled over and threatened to call the cops, because one of the guys was screaming at his wife, another was sobbing and talking about all the friends that had been killed overseas, and the rest of us were causing chaos. Bobbie assured the driver that this is what all of them had to go through every day, and she managed to regain control by telling everyone on board to sit down and put their hands on their laps.

It helped having people around me, but there were points where Bobbie ran out of patience and was sick of my behavior. She finally had me back after months away, and had endured multiple phone calls where she thought I wouldn't be coming home, but instead of having a happy father and husband, she had an absent Marine. I wish I could remember what we were arguing about when she one day gave me an ultimatum.

"If you want to be miserable all the time, then you can be miserable by yourself. I am taking Ethan out for a doctor's appointment, and when we come back we are going to leave and stay with my parents in Pennsylvania."

She left, and I didn't think she would come back. The thoughts of Shanfield and Walters and that IED blast circled around my head again, and that's when I thought to myself: *You know what—fuck it all.* I'd witnessed Marines die from alcohol poisoning on base, and figured it would be the best way to die. I raided our liquor cabinet and found two one-liter bottles of Milagro tequila. I wrote her a letter saying sorry, sent text messages to my friends that my wife had left me, and just started drinking as fast as I could. Within minutes of the first shot I was already throwing up, but I just kept going. It didn't matter by that point. My mind was made up and I was going to finish the job. I'd had enough. Between every few sips came Shanfield and Walters, the metal detector, the blast, the men around me in the hospital beds, and the feeling of guilt that wouldn't stop. This was the only option to stop the pain and the brain injuries making my life a living hell. Bobbie was an hour away with Ethan and had no idea why her phone kept ringing.

Like the day in 2008 with the sniper shot and the explosion just a few months before, I plunged into darkness. Was that it? Had I finished the job? Would I stop feeling pain? I suddenly woke up and realized I was sitting upright, and someone had strapped my head to the fridge with duct tape. I was panicking. I had no idea what was happening and no clue who had tied me down. I tried to look around but couldn't move. Bobbie had come home and found me passed out outside the bathroom floor and couldn't wake me, so she had called my best friend Dustin Bohde, next door. He was a corpsman with the 2nd battalion, 10th Marines, so he always had medical equipment on him, knowing he could be called to deal with a situation at any time. He somehow got me to vomit so he could get all of the tequila out of my system, and then stuck an IV line into each arm. By the time I woke up, the bags had almost run out of saline solution. Dustin saw my eyes had opened and kept telling me I was a dumbass, but I could see in his face that he was happy he got there in time to save me.

He saved my life. If it hadn't been for him, I wouldn't be here. Dustin understood my actions, but it was his duty to save me.

On October 1, 2010, I was promoted from Sergeant to Staff Sergeant, despite my condition, and despite all that had happened to put my career in limbo. It was an immensely proud moment for me to make one of the biggest jumps in ranks in the Marines, and a welcome break from the endless consultations and talks with doctors. It was recognition of the brushes with death, the endless gun battles, and the sleepless nights. Bobbie came to the ceremony at Camp Lejeune to pin the new ranks on my uniform, before a First Sergeant called me into his office to give me my first assignment. He shook my hand, congratulated me on the promotion, and told me I was the battalion's new SACO (Substance Abuse Control Officer)—the Marine in charge of handling urine samples and making sure colleagues stayed away from booze if they'd been involved in an incident related to alcohol. In my opinion I had been given a job that wasn't real leadership, especially after getting a promotion that was a huge honor to me, and I let the First Sergeant know I was furious with the new position. He tried to reassure me, and said: "This isn't any reflection on you. But you are the only Staff Sergeant on limited duty right now, and that is the position that needs filling." I had to check to make sure piss tests weren't corrupted or swapped with other liquids, and have meetings with anyone accused of substance abuse. I looked grown men in the eye while they dropped their pants and urinated in a cup.

I was a SACO for three weeks and hated it as much as being a recruiter. I told a new First Sergeant I would do anything to get out of it. He told me there was a chance I could go back to Coronado to help at the scout swimmers school, where I could use my experience from my beach raid training, and live in paradise on the West Coast. But there was a sudden U-turn—I was informed I would be sent to the Field Medical School in Camp Johnston, Florida, where the corpsman prepared for their deployments. I was told they couldn't afford to fly me across the country, and there was a spot that needed filling. I was mad again that I was being bumped into the roles that no one wanted, because I was recently promoted and on limited duty. On the other hand, I needed to follow orders, and I was happy I would no longer have to carry around urine samples.

One of the first people I spoke to when I arrived at Camp Johnston was a gunnery sergeant from Shanfield and Walter's battalion, who I last saw in Marjah the day before the blast. I flashed back to that fateful day again and was petrified he would hold their deaths against me, but he didn't. He was professional, and sent me on to go and meet the students I would be training.

I had no idea what my job was, or what I was doing as a brand-new staff sergeant who had been given the responsibility of making sure these new Marines were physically fit enough to do the job. I was warned to act like a pissed-off platoon sergeant at the start of their classes, but to be relaxed with them by the time they graduated. It was a major adjustment, because my natural reaction to any Marine was to be the meanest bastard I could. That was my sense of humor, and I knew that would get them prepared for the most unforgiving colleagues and the grim, relentless realities of the front line.

The students were doing immediate action drills on the first day, in which they responded to an IED attack and got into a gunfight with the enemy in close quarters. They had to mirror a combat scenario even though they were shooting blanks, and I was going to be harsh on anyone who got it wrong. I saw one of the students firing rounds at one of the Marines in front of him, and I switched gears to become a harsh instructor by running up to the shooter and kicking him in the Kevlar until he hit the ground. I was furious because he had just killed one of his own in friendly fire.

I started screaming at him: "You just shot your man. You killed him." Then I realized the shooter was a woman. I was already out of my element because I had rarely worked with women in training, and started to consider whether I had overreacted. The chief instructor watched this unfold, and started laughing so hard he had tears in his eyes.

"Bee," he said. "You aren't gonna last a week here. We can't curse at these students, we can't smoke in front of them, and we can't even have energy drinks near them. And you just kicked a female in the back and started screaming at her." I still didn't think I'd done anything wrong, and I couldn't seem to adjust to my new surroundings. It took less than three weeks for me to cement my reputation among the students as brutally honest, almost to the point I was a complete asshole.

It was a Friday night when one of the students came up to me while I was on duty, and said one of the Marines was talking about killing themselves. Considering what I was going through myself, and knowing how hard it was to get anyone to talk through their problems, I wanted to help. He said he was having issues with his girlfriend back home, and was stressed by the classes where the instructors were shouting and screaming every five minutes. I decided to give him some tough love and be as direct as I could. I knew too many Marines who had killed themselves after each of my deployments. Every time we got home, losing at least two guys was a certainty because the war and the life they came back to was too much. What he would experience and see was only going to get worse, and I wanted him to realize that relationship problems were insignificant. An average of twenty veterans a day were dying of suicide, and families were being destroyed beyond repair by the War on Terror.

"Dude, you were talking about killing yourself over a girl," I said. "That is the dumbest thing I have heard in my life. You've got to be the weakest person I've ever met. If you're going to kill yourself, do that shit outside so none of my students have to clean it up." The young student looked at me and walked away, and I made sure someone in the platoon kept an eye on him that night. My approach could have been gentler, but all I wanted to do was help. I wanted him to know that concerns about his girlfriend would seem insignificant when he was deployed. Being direct was the only way I thought I could get through to him. Maybe I was channeling some of my own frustrations, but he needed to be ready to face the reality of being away from home, before he finished training. I somehow managed to escape disciplinary action for my callous speech.

The self-medication through drinking continued with the sergeants around me who had experienced the same level of combat in Helmand Province and Iraq. We worked the students to their limits and gave them the best training possible during the day, but when it was time to clock off, we hit the bars together to relieve the stress. My company commanders had no idea how much we drank, because they distanced themselves from the instructors' lives. They didn't realize how much of an impact my alcoholism was having on me until we were on a six-mile hike with the students. Those who failed to complete the distance wouldn't become corpsmen, a relief to those who wanted to be X-ray specialists or dental technicians on an aircraft carrier. They hadn't been exposed to the stress I had during bootcamp, and didn't have to carry heavy packs during their physical fitness tests. My idea of training was more ruthless; while I looked at a six-mile hike as a joke, they were absolutely terrified. A girl who was carrying one of the sixty-pound packs, and couldn't have weighed more than ninety pounds, started falling behind and slowing down the rest of the group. I was getting angry, and during one of our rest breaks, I went over to give her one of my lectures.

"You're weak. You are keeping everybody behind you. If you're going to fail, then just get on the truck and fail. I don't care." She rolled her eyes at me when I finished, so I picked her up with one hand on each side of her Kevlar vest, and threw her off the side of the road. I was screaming in her face with such rage that I didn't know what I was saying, and I was ready to beat the crap out of her, when a hand touched my shoulder and pulled me back. It was the commanding sergeant, and I knew I was in serious trouble that could get me kicked out. After everything I had been through, and all my deployments, it would be one of my ridiculous outbursts that could bring an end to the career I had wanted since I was a Boy Scout.

I walked into the training office expecting a verbal dressing down from the company commander, similar to the one I had just given the girl. He handed me a letter with a Non-Punitive Letter of Caution (NPLOC), which stated that I had performed my duties carelessly and to make sure I exercised greater care in the future. He then made me an offer: "This can go on your service record, or it will disappear if you talk to someone about what you are going through."

I needed help, and it almost took getting kicked out for me to properly address it. But I had a second chance, and I made sure the students got the best training possible in between our partying sessions. I was proud to be teaching these young men and women everything I knew, and my asshole teaching techniques seemed to pay off. A couple of years after I finished at Camp Johnson, I got a handwritten letter from one of the corpsmen who was working on a base when a mortar exploded during a training exercise. There were multiple casualties, and he managed to treat eight Marines in the space of just a few minutes by giving them tourniquets and checking them over. In his note he thanked me and the other instructors, saying that if we hadn't been in his face and screaming at him, he would not have been prepared for that dire situation and wouldn't have been able to save lives. It felt good knowing that—despite my unorthodox leadership—these Marines were ready to give the level of care I had received on the battlefield, and were primed to look after and try to save men like Cooper, Dunn, Shanfield, and Walters. I felt like it would go a small way to make up for some of the casualties I was responsible for.

CHAPTER 15

When I was selected to become a suicide prevention master trainer in the middle of 2012, I had to laugh at the irony of trying to take my own life with two bottles of tequila. They sent me to the school two weeks after shouting at the young sailor who wanted to kill himself. I'm sure it wasn't a coincidence. The brain fog, angry flare-ups, and flashbacks were still dominating my life and my personality, and my mind was still out in Afghanistan, crouched in trenches and under heavy Taliban gunfire.

I was chosen to train other people how to not kill themselves, and it was an enormous wake-up call, urging me to adapt to my brain injuries and open up about my suffering. The suicide master prevention training was new to the Marines, and a battalion would have to take a class every six months to prevent suicidal thoughts like mine. The start of the course presented me with an opportunity that I didn't believe I would ever be comfortable with.

I was sitting in a classroom in a circle with twenty male and female Marine instructors, all looking at each other. The topic of conversation could have easily been beer, motorbikes, fighting sports, or guns. Instead, we had to be at our most emotionally vulnerable and give examples from our lives where we considered ending it all. Some grunts found this impossible, but other Marines started talking about hardships they had faced in their lives.

Screw it, I thought to myself. I hadn't talked to anyone about what I was going through, only Bobbie and a couple of my friends knew about the tequila incident, and this was an opportunity to open up. I described helping recruit Shanfield, the times I met his family, us reuniting in Marjah, the day of the IED, and all the times I had thought about him since. I told the group I was responsible for putting him in that building and how it should have been me in a casket on the flight back from Helmand Province. I ended with how the anger, depression, and alienation became so overwhelming I tried to drink myself to death, and ended up with my neighbor duct-taping my head to my fridge. I had to stop a couple of times because I started to choke up. You could hear a pin drop as everyone in the class just stared at me, and a wave of relief rushed over me that I hadn't felt in months. I felt I could open up to the class, because it was likely I would never see them again and none of what I said would be reported. When I finished the speech, the instructor told the group to take a break. The Marine up next said there was no way he could follow me. There was still a mammoth road ahead for me to get anywhere close to normal, but I realized that my brutal honesty could help me.

Before the class, I started seeing a civilian doctor who talked to me like I was a normal person—unlike the medical personnel in the infantry unit, who were more concerned about whether you were battle ready, and didn't have time to go through your emotional problems. He told me that the thoughts I was having weren't normal, and was the first to change my perception of PTSD. I assumed that the main symptoms of depression were going internal and being quiet and weepy, but he assured me that it manifested itself in many different forms, including the anger and aggression I was experiencing. I started to understand that my traumatic brain injuries and physiological reactions in my head could be driving my intense reactions, and it got me to take my treatment more seriously. For the first time, I felt like someone was taking me seriously, and that it was acceptable to have a conversation about the mental issues that for so long had come with a stigma attached. The Marines had many struggles with psychological treatment, including programs where the psychiatrists would spend most of their time discussing whether the sessions were covered by health insurance.

It was during my treatment—towards the end of 2012— that I figured out I would never be fit to lead an infantry platoon as a sergeant, and began to consider my options. I would forget simple things when doing paperwork, I was still getting lost, and my anger issues still wouldn't subside. If administrative duties stressed me out, there was no way I would be able to lead men into another situation like Garmsir or Marjah, and my friends started talking about wanting to get out. They were done with the Marines.

And so was I, it seemed: the Marines announced they had too many staff sergeants, and would be using an algorithm based on years of service to determine who would stay and who would go. But I was also told I would never again be deployed. I wanted to go back to Afghanistan, or get the chance to fight with my buddies in Iraq, and kept telling my senior officers there was nothing wrong with me, but the stark reality was that I couldn't lead Marines into combat anymore. It would be a struggle to survive. The dream career—that began as a fantasy while running around Ohio cornfields—was coming to an end, with me getting violently sick after running only a few hundred yards, forgetting what I had for breakfast, and getting lost in grocery stores. Bobbie and I got into furious arguments about my future. While I was drinking one night, I started yelling at her like I was a staff sergeant and she a boot. I had to leave the house to prevent myself doing something stupid, so I ran into our yard and launched Ethan's plastic slide against a wall.

The decision to leave was made easier by the options I was given for what would have been my next orders, after I requested a deployment on either the East or West Coast, or in Hawaii. The monitor in charge of determining where I would go next told me I had never been stationed overseas, so the next destination would be abroad.

"What the hell? I have been to Afghanistan four times and probably spent a total of three years over there. What do you mean?" I snapped back at him.

"But you have never been 'stationed' overseas," he responded, trying his best to explain the difference. "We have a position open for you that I think would be perfect, and we need to send you. It's in Greenland."

"Have you lost your goddamn mind?" I said. *I am not dealing with the extreme cold. At this point of my career, I am only going somewhere warm, like Jamaica,* I thought to myself. He tried to sweeten the deal by insisting Bobbie and Ethan could come with me. I said no, so then they offered me another stint as a recruiter, and that was another *hell no.* My mind was made up, and I told Bobbie that on our seventh wedding anniversary, April 1, 2012, I would be leaving the Marines.

I filled out my paperwork, and the voluntary separation pay algorithm based on my years of service determined a payout of $103,000, which came to roughly $87,000 after taxes. Training exercises and military briefings were soon replaced by sessions teaching me how to write a resume, financial planning, and how to adapt our language to civilian life—because there were things we said in combat and in barracks that were far from appropriate.

I was also told I could apply for disability benefits with Veterans Affairs, which I hadn't realized was a possibility until my service ended and I needed it—as a former grunt, I would soon be broke if I didn't get a job. If I could prove my problems were caused by my work as a Marine, I was entitled to compensation. A Veteran Services Officer told me he could help. He said, "We'll start with your head and make our way down. If there is something wrong with you that wasn't an issue when you joined, we can make a claim to the VA."

I had nine doctor's appointments in three days, and underwent a series of tests so the VA could do their own assessments. The tests were more intense than anything I had experienced in Landstuhl. My neuropsychology exam was two days of two-dimensional and three-dimensional puzzles mixed with memory exercises, where I had to remember certain words and numbers. They made me play games where I had to put pegs in holes the size of toothpicks, and I noticed my hands would shake so much I couldn't finish. It was a tremor I didn't know I had. They were tasks four-year-old children could complete, but I couldn't. I was furious that I was incapable of doing the simplest assignments, but it helped me realize the severity of my problems.

When all the tests were over, the doctor called Bobbie and me into his office. He was able to tell me which parts of my brain were damaged, how it had happened, why it meant I was unable to perform certain functions, and how it was causing the memory fogs and the vivid flashbacks. There were physiological causes that went far beyond the issues caused by my PTSD. I felt vindicated, because everything started to add up and I was getting a more complete picture of my health problems.

A psychiatrist contracted by the VA then called me in, and said he wanted to know everything that had happened since joining up. I went beyond what I'd talked about in the suicide prevention master training, and was completely honest about everything in my career, from Shanfield and Walters, to my guilt, my drinking, my rage, my problems socializing, my flashbacks, and my PTSD.

I finished my story and said with a smile: "So, doctor, do you think I am nuts?"

He laughed and told me, "I have a diagnosis, but I have only been contracted by the VA, so I can't tell you the results before they get my file. All my conclusions and recommendations are on this computer screen. I am going to leave you alone while I go outside for a cigarette."

With a sly grin on his face as he reached the door to leave his office, he turned and said, "Whatever you do, don't look at the computer screen." I got the hint, went to sit in his chair, and moved the computer mouse so I could see documents on display.

I read the top line and saw something I had never heard before: "Dissociative Rage Disorder." It was also known as "Intermittent Explosive Disorder," the symptoms of which included sudden outbursts of anger and violence, without being provoked and with no apparent reason. I was grateful I could finally put a name—and give an explanation—to the illness that was causing me problems with Bobbie, Ethan, my family, and my friends, and had contributed to me being unfit to continue with the Marines. I had a case for compensation, and I finally had the confirmation that what I was feeling wasn't solely psychological.

Despite my progress, the problems persisted. I started seeing another psychiatrist at the VA who clearly wasn't interested in my problems, and wouldn't pay attention when I talked. There were also language barriers because English wasn't her first language, which was concerning as she was responsible for prescribing my medication. The problems started from the first appointment, when she would refer to unrelated parts of my career and ask me bizarre questions that were inaccurate or weren't relevant.

"So, what year did you get caught up with the IED in Cuba?"

"What are you talking about," I'd say back: "The IED was in 2010, and I was in Cuba in 2003. I didn't even get shot at."

"Oh, sorry about that. So, who is this Little Man you keep mentioning and who you keep hallucinating about?" "Little Man" was the nickname I had for Ethan.

I was given a Total and Permanent Disability designation, which meant I was entitled to full benefits and my condition had no chance of improving. My mood swings and outbursts were still frequent, and even though I was now taking a shopping list of prescription medication, I was still having issues with the VA. I had a diagnosis after a multitude of tests, but no real treatment program to try and remedy my issues.

Six months after I started receiving benefits checks, I came home to find Bobbie in the kitchen staring at me with fury.

"What did you do?" she said to me, while holding a letter from the VA that said I would stop receiving my disability payments because of the $88,000 separation payout from the Marines. The checks would cease until my compensation credits hit the same amount. I had erroneously thought it was a one-off that we could use to pay off all our loans and bills, and give me a cushion while I didn't have an income. The pause in my benefits also meant Bobbie and Ethan stopped getting access to insurance, so I had to find a job, despite a diagnosis that stated I couldn't work.

I didn't know what to do. I couldn't fight, and my brain injuries meant I couldn't go back to college. My resume listed one job since I was seventeen. But I remembered all the time I had spent as a bookworm at school. I thought about all the classes that had helped me transition into civilian life when I got out of the Marines, and I thought about all the time I had spent shouting at Marines in a classroom myself. I decided I would now try my hand at teaching veterans in my position. I wanted to help those leaving the military who had a multitude of physical and mental problems, and who didn't know how to apply for benefits, find classes, or try and start a normal life.

In April 2013, I handed out resumes and got a call from Calibre Systems, which had a contract with the Veterans Benefits Administration to teach compulsory classes for members of the military getting out. During my second interview with Mark Toll—a Marine who got up to Lieutenant Colonel—he asked me why I had left so early, because I was only thirty-two and it was rare for Staff Sergeants to not work all the way until their twenty-year retirement. He didn't believe me when I said, "It was my time" and "It just wasn't the right fit," so I said, "Sir, just google my name." We kept talking for another two minutes when he interrupted and shouted, "Holy shit! I've seen that picture."

"I am getting out because that is not the only time I have been hit during deployment, and my wife was done," I said with a laugh, and he ended up giving me a job as an assistant site leader covering three bases in North Carolina for $27,000 a year. All of my colleagues were messed up by our service in some way, and we connected with stories of who we knew, who we lost, our gunfights, and how we had been trying to recover. I taught classes during my schedule of constant medical appointments, and learned firsthand the pitfalls of the VA bureaucracy. The doctors and nurses gave every one of their patients their highest standard of care, but they faced constant setbacks with their resources stretched thin.

Despite the problems, I got to do what I loved: helping veterans like me and sharing stories about what we'd been through. I bonded with the men and women who came into my classrooms with my dull PowerPoint presentations. I showed them YouTube videos to lighten the mood and joked with them about the stupid stuff I had done in Afghanistan. I was given a book an inch-and-a-half thick full of all the benefits these service members could get, and I had to memorize them all. The bullish teaching style I picked up during recruitment service and Field Medical Training got me into trouble when I cursed, but most of the people in my class would just laugh, and when I got belligerent or my memory issues played up they would understand. I urged those who would listen to push for compensation for every injury or sickness they developed, and I would always say: "The beautiful thing about us Marines is we are more fucked up than we think we are. We were hit with more shit than anyone in the military, and you deserve the money if something is wrong with you."

It was the beginning of 2014 when I started to get even more frustrated with our management at the Calibre annual training event in Washington D.C., with instructors from across the country. We were in a hotel for a seminar when Deputy Under Secretary for Benefits Rosye Cloud came on stage to do a speech praising our hard work. She stunned me when she said: "No veteran should have to worry about making less than $30,000 a year." When she finished and asked if there were any questions, I put up my hand and caused everyone to turn their heads and glare. They all wanted to leave, and I was slowing down their trip back to the bar.

"Hey ma'am," I said. "I'm William Bee, and I'm the assistant site lead from Camp Lejeune, and I'm teaching classes for veterans across three bases. I'm making $27,000 a year. I can't tell my friends because they would laugh at me." The room fell silent and she stared at me for a few moments, before giving a vague response I wish I could remember, but that set the tone for the next five years in the job. I stayed there because I didn't think I was qualified to do anything else: it was secure and the alternative was stacking shelves in Walmart, which was daunting, because my head injuries often meant I got lost in the aisles while shopping with Bobbie and Ethan. More defense contractors came in and made it clear our role was to teach as many people as we could, and increase the quotas of classes we were running every day, because it meant more money. They didn't care about us or the veterans they were serving—they were focused on their calculators, spreadsheets, and pocketbooks.

The only thing that kept me sane were the days when people from all branches of the military would walk into my office and ask for help planning the rest of their lives. Most of them had no idea what they were going to do when they got out, and wanted to know how to get a degree or use their benefits. I got to tell them they would be getting $1,500 this month, and the VA would pay their tuition if they wanted to go to school, and I would witness the moment they recognized that their hard work and sacrifice could still pay off. In between classes, I went online and completed computer courses for myself that helped the wounded get back to work, and my friends who did the same went on to high-end jobs in top companies like Cisco. I watched these life-changing events with pride, though the battle I was fighting at home didn't let up. Like in Marjah, it seemed like I woke up to another firefight every morning, but there was no one shooting at me. It was all in my head.

CHAPTER 16

It was the winter of 2014, and Bobbie and I were fighting all the time. The drinking hadn't stopped, and the nightmares with flashbacks of the blast, Shanfield, and Walters were constant. Not an hour would go by without me thinking about sending them into that building, and feeling the guilt of their deaths all over again. My hallucinations were so severe I would hear Bobbie or Ethan calling out for me, even if they weren't at home, and I would suddenly smell a smoke grenade or feel the heat of the Afghanistan sun while standing in the middle of a store.

Bobbie couldn't sleep in a separate room to avoid my rage and violent flashbacks, because I would sleepwalk, and she needed to keep track of me. She went back to my Marine command begging to get me help so she could protect herself, and was simply told to hide any weapons we had behind a locked wooden door, similar to those I'd spent three years kicking down to get into mud buildings in Afghanistan. I would have no problem getting my hands on something dangerous if I tried. Luckily, we didn't have any guns in the house.

The list of powerful antipsychotics I was being prescribed had increased to eighteen pills to take every day. I lined the opioids up on the table and popped them one by one, in a ritual more natural than breakfast. There was a bottle for depression, another for seizures, one to help me sleep, another for panic attacks, one for anxiety, another for low testosterone, and medication for ulcers. The list was endless and included Vicodin, the highly addictive painkiller I had been given after the accident in the water during training.

The drugs the VA loaded me up on, while I waited to see a doctor or specialist, horrified Bobbie, and she would spend hours online researching the side effects to make sure I was safe. She was scrolling through and found that Sumatriptan Succinate, the pill I took to help ease my migraines, could kill me if I mixed it with other drugs including Paroxetine, which was on my shopping list of prescriptions. A cocktail of the two medications could cause my serotonin levels to increase to the point it was fatal. I got stomach problems, and would spend hours throwing up in the bathroom because of the pills that were doing untold damage to my body. Bobbie told my doctors she refused to let me take them, but they kept filling out scripts believing it would help me mask my suffering, when all it did was make it worse. The staff thought I could fend for myself with this magical collection of pill bottles. What shocked me even more, was that I found out almost sixty-eight thousand veterans in VA care were addicted to opioids at the time, and many because of over-prescription.

The prescription problems manifested themselves in the most tragic way with sniper Rob Richards, who'd grown to be one of my closest friends in Jacksonville after he was medically retired by the Marines. The constant publicity around the 2012 video, and the injuries from the IED, took an enormous toll on his life with depression, PTSD, and excruciating pain that left him bedridden for weeks—and the VA used medication to help him cope. He was found dead in his home from drug toxicity in November 2014, when he was just twenty-eight years old. He was taking twelve prescriptions, and started self-medicating with heroin and steroids to try and cover up the scars of combat. His wife Rachel, one of our closest friends, had watched him get and stay clean for six months, but it wasn't enough. When he was interred in Arlington, I wanted his legacy to be one of the best scout snipers in the business, not one ruined by upper command abandoning you over a video or by a death that no veteran deserves. He was cremated, and Rachel put his ashes in an ammo can bearing his name, the scout sniper motto ("One shot, one kill"), and a quote from Ernest Hemmingway that read: "There is no hunting like the hunting of man, and those who have hunted armed men long enough and liked it, never care for anything else thereafter." Members of the American Infidels Motorcycle

Club, who helped Richards and his family, joined the mourners to pay their respects. They were his brothers, and I go to the ride they hold in his memory every year.

For Bobbie, it was like she had two toddlers, me and Ethan. Between my return from Germany and 2014, our house turned into a gallery of post-it notes and lists with tasks and instructions, because my memory was still failing me. I had to be supervised when cooking. I wasn't getting better, and I knew my brain would never heal. I kept imagining what it would be like if I went back overseas to fight alongside my buddies. I would get excited, and then I would realize it was never going to happen. Before 2010, I was outgoing and socialized with my friends, but Bobbie now struggled to get me out of the house, unless my day was planned out in an itinerary.

Weed was the only thing that actually helped. I first smoked cannabis in the winter of 2014, after an appointment with a psychiatrist. For an hour she made me go through the most traumatic moments of my time as a Marine, laid out a suggested treatment plan, and then said: "I really shouldn't be saying this, but I wish I could prescribe you cannabis." I ended up smoking with my neighbor and we sat, laughed, and watched TV. I saw an infomercial for blue-light-blocking glasses and thought it was going to change the face of the earth, so I figured I'd had too much, but it made me relaxed and gave me an escape.

Cannabis stopped my nightmares and dark thoughts, so I started lighting up a pipe twenty minutes before bed, to get a peaceful night's sleep, like I used to get before my first trip to Garmsir. It worked better than the medication the VA was giving me, and I wasn't being an angry asshole to Bobbie, or flying off the handle at the smallest spark. I dropped some of the prescriptions and my health started improving, and when the VA asked if I was smoking, I never lied. I smoked with my and Bobbie's parents and started referring to it as my medicine. I needed to be more mellow for my family, and I shouldn't have had to rely on marijuana to make me feel normal, while I was still struggling to get regular help for my traumatic brain injuries. Even while I was working with the Veterans Benefits Administration, I was being caught up in a backlog, and forced to wait days and sometimes weeks to see or even talk to someone. Bobbie was the only person I could truly talk to. My four-eleven angel was the last line of defense keeping me alive, and she tried to keep me on course when I started to drift, but there was only so much she could take.

2015 was when I received the letter from Wills Robinson, asking me to do the article for DailyMail.com. Like I said before, I was reluctant to talk to someone who had no idea what it was like to face the Taliban and watch their friends die. Wills was a British journalist living in New York; how could he possibly relate to my issues? But my family told me it was time to get my story out there, so people could understand what we went through, and what we still go through, and they were right. The article came out, and suddenly doors opened I thought had been closed for good. Around this time, Bobbie was still fighting to get me the Purple Heart that so many others in my squad had received, in addition to fighting to get me medically retired. Wills Robinson's story prompted an investigation into why I hadn't received the Purple Heart.

A few days after the article came out, I got a phone call from the VA saying they had been "directed" to get in touch with me, to get me some treatment. I couldn't help but laugh and said: "I've been wanting a phone call from you guys for a while." From my first appointment with them, I stressed that I needed to see a psychiatrist, but instead had been cast aside and left to be treated by my general physician. They assigned me a new case manager and finally directed me to a head specialist who would go beyond the headshaking and memory tests I had been through with no improvement. It was ridiculous that it took a story about my struggles on a news website to get me the help I needed. I told my students that it proved how bad their access to doctors and essential care could get, because not every veteran had a journalist wanting to write about them.

The same month the article came out, I got a call from Dr. Tania Glenn, inviting my family to her office in Cedar Park, Texas, which was dedicated to helping veterans and first responders deal with PTSD. She saw the article and reached out to Bobbie, because she wanted to try and help with EMDR (Eye Movement Desensitization And Reprocessing). I had never heard of the technique and dismissed it as hypnotism when I looked it up, but when she sent me some articles on the benefits, and referenced other veterans she had helped, I decided to fly down and give it a try, because nothing else had worked.

In our sessions, like countless other times before, I recalled all the most traumatic moments of my career: my first gunfight, the sniper shot in 2008, holding Cooper's hand, telling Dunn he would be okay, Shanfield and Walters, the IED blast, my suicide attempt with tequila, and the endless nightmares, memory losses, and fits of rage. While I went through my tragic list, she waved her finger and shined lights into my eyes, watching for moments when my pupils would shift or get wider, and every time she noticed an intense response, she got me to keep talking to figure out what was setting me off. It seemed like a Jedi mind trick and each session gave me a screaming migraine, but I wanted to persist and see it would pay off.

At night, Dr. Glenn's Peer Support Case Manager Steven Thornhill—an Army veteran who had served in Iraq—would take me into Austin, into areas that would normally send me into a spiral, and share our stories that had traumatized us both. Each neighborhood we chose was more crowded than the last, and on our last night we headed downtown to the bars on Sixth Street that were packed full of people. I didn't get agitated, I didn't panic, and I didn't feel any violent urges as I squeezed myself down the busy sidewalks. Watching and listening to Steven gave me confidence that I could control my life, and try to get back some of the traits that had made me an outgoing, loveable guy before 2012. By the end of the week, I was able to walk down the street in Austin, in a rush of people during lunch, without breaking down. I was never going to be able to turn off my PTSD—I would be stuck with it for the rest of my life—but I could cope, and try to make myself better for the sake of my family.

After years of Bobbie fighting and trying to get together the right paperwork, I was awarded the Purple Heart in August, which is rare for someone with traumatic brain injuries. The symptoms of a TBI are often invisible, and sometimes aren't considered to be serious. To receive a Purple Heart, you also have to prove the wounds were caused by the enemy, and problems with my records, and the difficulty of linking my injuries directly to the IED blast, made it harder to get me approved. As they pinned the medal on me at the No Man Left Behind monument at Camp Lejeune, in front of my wife and son, a tear rolled down my cheek. It was recognition for multiple IEDs blowing out my eardrums from a wall four feet away. It was bittersweet because—like every other day—I had a moment where I could see Shanfield and Walters' faces, and told myself I was the reason they were there too. It was so emotional because the medal signified a legacy I could pass on to my son. I can tell him how important it is to serve our amazing country, and also explain the sacrifices it entails. When he turns eighteen and considers putting on the uniform, he will know the dangers I went through.

In 2017, Bobbie, Ethan and I started to grow out of our cookie-cutter neighborhood in Jacksonville where every house had the same color scheme, like in a scene from *The Stepford Wives*. We saw the same people every day, and the routine of living so close to the base that had dominated my life was tiring. Living so close to base didn't help my constant reminders of Shanfield, Walters, Cooper, and Dunn. After eight years in the Marines—with three in combat—I had already missed so much of Ethan's childhood and being a part of what he was doing at school, that I wanted to enjoy spending time with him in a place with more freedom. Bobbie and I still had bumps in our relationships—there was drinking, and the place we thought was home had bad vibes.

So we took the initiative and moved to a new house in Jacksonville, with woods in the backyard that were a spitting image of what Kristan and I used to play in as children, when we were kicked out of the trailer. It was a place where we could walk around the neighborhood and Ethan could run and play in the streets. There was a pool and a dock where I could take him fishing for the afternoon, but we would never catch anything. I stood in awe as my "Little Guy" battled his special needs from second grade all the way to trying out for his junior high basketball team. Bobbie was happier and our marriage started to get better. She used the sociology degree she studied for, while caring for Ethan and me, to start caring for the elderly and children who'd been through trauma. Like me, she wanted to help people who needed it the most and teach them that there is always hope.

I stuck with my teaching job at the VBA until 2019, when the bureaucracy started to distract from me giving veterans a better life. I wasn't happy. I was sick of sitting behind a desk waiting for a phone to ring, for $27,000 a year. My psychiatric record stopped me from considering joining the police, and I didn't like the sound of private security, or sitting in an oil field in Saudi Arabia as a contractor, so I started dropping off my resumes at any company with links to the military of security roles I could think of.

One day in 2019, I went to a veteran's career fair at Camp Lejeune, and saw a stand surrounded by robots dressed in uniform. The stand was for Marathon Targets, and they were advertising jobs working on a live-fire range, where Marines shot at motorized targets that would dart across the battlefield like the Taliban, and flee when we opened fire. I didn't think there was a chance in hell of getting what I thought could be the coolest career—operating robots used for grunt target practice. But I handed in an application after talking with Pete Burns, another Marine who invaded Afghanistan in 2001.

I was in Ethan's doctor's office, where he was getting a physical to clear him to play basketball, when I got the call that I got the job to work with the robots and the lasers. I was floored because my resume was still limited, but it meant I never had to sit and work in a cubicle again, but could keep helping the military. I would be back to spending most of my time outdoors like I did as a child, and the guns I would be playing with were a bit bigger and more powerful. My desire to serve had never died, and I could be close to the sounds of gunfights and Marines screaming at each other, that I missed. Pushing aside my close calls with death, the trauma, and the PTSD, I never forgot the times I spent with my best friends battling on the other side of the world.

CHAPTER 17

Union Cemetery in Cambria County, Pennsylvania, is a beautiful and quiet place on a stretch of lawn by the side of a country road. The entrance is across from a wooden barn with an angled roof and red door. It is well kept and surrounded by cornfields like my childhood home in rural Ohio. There is a white chapel, only a few headstones, and cars rarely drive by. It is also the final resting place of twenty-two-year-old Derek Lee Shanfield. The cemetery is just a twenty-minute drive from where Bobbie's parents live, but it took me a while to find the courage to visit his grave. Shanfield's mom told me his death wasn't my fault and insisted I tell her whenever I decided to lay flowers, but I couldn't get over it. After his funeral in 2010, I sat down with his parents and went through that life-altering day in Marjah, in detail. I was honest about everything that happened, and why I was responsible for him being inside that building with walls rigged with IEDs. I explained why I was the reason his remains were picked up in trash bags, and flown home in a coffin draped in the American flag. His mother insisted I was not to blame, but she couldn't change my mind.

I finally plucked up the courage to go and visit on Thanksgiving in 2015, and now I go to the grave at least twice a year. I stand there alone with excruciating guilt. Not an hour goes by that I don't think about Shanfield—the kid who was contemplating a career in the Marines when I first met him as a young high school student—and Walters, both twenty-two-year-olds who had so much of their lives still to give. Every time I stand there, I reflect and remind myself that I am not the only veteran in this position.

I have still not been medically retired by the Marines. The VA declared me 100 percent disabled and gave me benefits, but in the eyes of the military, there wasn't enough evidence to prove I was too wounded to carry on being a Marine. I was put on limited duty, told I wasn't healthy enough to be deployed, and I knew I wasn't able to lead a platoon. My PTSD and rage disorder made me a liability. Even though I was broken and knew my brain would never heal, I continued to give it my all. I didn't want my injuries to define me, so I kept performing well in my physical tests and made it clear I still wanted to fight. I wanted to go back to the battlefield; there was just no way I could. If I had completely given up my dream of joining my friends to fight again, I may have been retired and given the full package of benefits that come with it. Now we have a team of lawyers taking the government to court to fight my case.

I am trying to help myself come to terms with my life, and increase the understanding of what thousands of Marines and ex-servicemen and women go through, not just in the United States but around the world. I want to be clear: some troops get good treatment, some don't even need it and don't seek it. But far too often, those in trouble are left to fend for themselves—and that often means they are forced into homelessness, a life of crime, or suicide. In June 2020—a decade after leaving Marjah—one of the Marines who fought alongside me on that fateful day and spent years grappling with the anguish, took his own life. His scars had never healed. He was thirty-seven years old, with a wife and seven-year-old son. His death hit me as hard as Cooper, Dunn, Shanfield, and Walters. He wasn't the first who decided life was too much, and he won't be the last.

Those photos of me were shared as an example of the bravery and sacrifice by Marines in the battlefield. I sacrificed everything for my country, and can only say I am brave some of the time. But even those images, and standing in the firing line of the world's most evil fighters, still didn't get me the help I needed. Some have good experiences with the VA and others simply don't need their care. Others struggle like me when it should be far easier. They should be able to get a doctor's appointment without waiting weeks, and should be given the decency of care after risking their lives thousands of miles away. It took ten years for me to finally build up the courage to tell my story and now I know, more than ever, that it is an experience that needs to be shared and understood. I'm not the only one. There are men and women who need help now, and there will be many more in the future. Every day is a battle, and it will be for generations.

I am back in my bedroom in Jacksonville, North Carolina, staring at the ceiling, with Bobbie at my side. There may still be nightmares, there may still be sleepwalking, and there may still be screaming. My son is sound asleep in the other room with his whole life in front of him, and one day I will sit him down and tell him everything, and hope he can see his daddy in the photo and be proud of how I defended my country with honor. Every day I spend at the range is a blessing, and keeps me connected to what I miss the most, fighting with some of the best men I will ever know. Some are still here, some aren't, and we will undoubtedly lose some more along the way. Those who I have lost will always be with me. What I have learned is that no matter how dark your life becomes, how grim your prognosis is, or how slow your recovery seems, there is always hope. Improvise, adapt, and overcome—that is the Marine mantra. It is what boots are first taught when they arrive at camp, it is what we use to fight our toughest battles, and it is a philosophy that I use every day.

My life is far from perfect, but with my angel and "Little Man" beside me, I can be optimistic there will be happier days. I look back at those photos and everything I brought home from my Afghanistan tours, and struggle to grasp everything that has happened since, and my brain injuries still sometimes make it hard to remember. But when I left the Marines, I didn't think my life could get any worse; now, I don't think it could get any better.

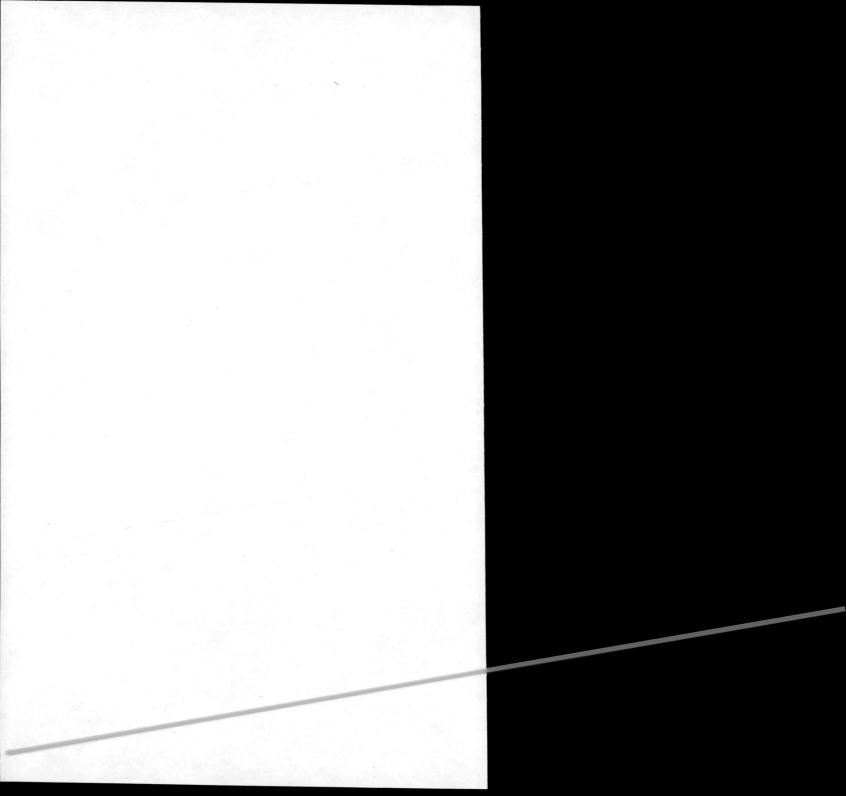